ABSOLUTE BEGINNER'S GUIDE

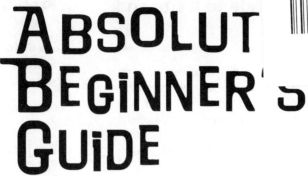

TO

a Lite and Healthy Lifestyle

Nicole Haywood, M.A., R.D.

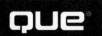

800 East 96th Street,
Indianapolis, Indiana 46240

Absolute Beginner's Guide to a Lite and Healthy Lifestyle

International Standard Book Number: 0-7897-3315-3

Library of Congress Catalog Card Number: 20044114913

Printed in the United States of America

First Printing: January 2005

08 07 06 05   4 3 2 1

Trademarks

All terms mentioned in this book that are known to be trademarks or service marks have been appropriately capitalized. Que Publishing cannot attest to the accuracy of this information. Use of a term in this book should not be regarded as affecting the validity of any trademark or service mark.

Warning and Disclaimer

Every effort has been made to make this book as complete and as accurate as possible, but no warranty or fitness is implied. The information provided is on an "as is" basis. The author and the publisher shall have neither liability nor responsibility to any person or entity with respect to any loss or damages arising from the information contained in this book.

Bulk Sales

Que offers excellent discounts on this book when ordered in quantity for bulk purchases or special sales. For more information, please contact

U.S. Corporate and Government Sales
1-800-382-3419
corpsales@pearsontechgroup.com

For sales outside of the U.S., please contact

International Sales
international@pearsoned.com

Executive Editor
Candace Hall

Development Editor
Sean Dixon

Managing Editor
Charlotte Clapp

Project Editor
Seth Kerney

Copy Editor
Geneil Breeze

Indexer
Erika Millen

Proofreader
Tonya Simpson

Publishing Coordinator
Cindy Teeters

Interior Designer
Anne Jones

Cover Designer
Dan Armstrong

Contents at a Glance

Think
Was this meal satisfied my psychological hunger?
Was this meal satisfied by physical hunger?

- Do I reward myself with food? - yes -
         give myself something
                  else instead.

- what triggers negative eating patterns?
                  What could be an
                           alternative?

= what do I gain if I don't reward myself
                  with food?

= what won't I gain if I don't reward
                  myself with food?

= Do I eat in response to internal or external
     cues?

Table of Contents

About the Author

Nicole Haywood is the Wellness Coordinator in the Center for Educational Services at the National Institute for Fitness and Sport (NIFS). Nicole is a registered dietitian and has a master's degree in Family and Consumer Sciences. She completed her Bachelor of Science in Dietetics at Purdue University, West Lafayette, Indiana, and her graduate work at Ball State University, Muncie, Indiana. At NIFS, she specializes in behavior modification and developing healthy eating attitudes and patterns. Nicole coordinates several weight management programs and develops and presents wellness lectures on nutrition, fitness, and wellness topics for corporate and community groups. She occasionally appears on Indianapolis radio and television programs to disseminate current health news for central Indiana residents. Nicole also provides individual nutrition consultations related to making healthy food choices, wellness, fitness, healthy body weight, eating disorders, and managing chronic health conditions.

Dedication

To my husband Joshua and to our families—it's a privilege to share this life with all of you.

Acknowledgments

This book would not have been possible without the help of many people, first and foremost, my amazing clients. You have shared your lives and experiences with me over the years and have contributed immeasurably to my philosophy and the content of this book. Special thanks to those of you who shared your personal stories that they might inspire others!

To Mom and Aunt Joanne; colleagues and friends Heather Hedrick, Amy Moyer, Jodi Hazard, and Suzanne Caithamer; interns Amy Speed-Andrews, Jennifer Titus, and Carly Mayers; and clients who prefer to remain anonymous—your feedback and encouragement through this whole process were invaluable! Thank you to everyone at Que and particularly Karen Whitehouse, Sean Dixon, Candace Hall, Seth Kerney, Geneil Breeze, and other behind-the-scenes staff for your patience, skill, and guidance. And most importantly, praise and thanks to God for the wonderful opportunities with which I've been blessed.

We Want to Hear from You!

As the reader of this book, *you* are our most important critic and commentator. We value your opinion and want to know what we're doing right, what we could do better, what areas you'd like to see us publish in, and any other words of wisdom you're willing to pass our way.

As an executive editor for Que Publishing, I welcome your comments. You can email or write me directly to let me know what you did or didn't like about this book—as well as what we can do to make our books better.

Please note that I cannot help you with technical problems related to the topic of this book. We do have a User Services group, however, where I will forward specific technical questions related to the book.

When you write, please be sure to include this book's title and author as well as your name, email address, and phone number. I will carefully review your comments and share them with the author and editors who worked on the book.

Email: feedback@quepublishing.com

Mail: Candace Hall
         Executive Editor
         Que Publishing
         800 East 96th Street
         Indianapolis, IN 46240 USA

For more information about this book or another Que title, visit our website at www.quepublishing.com. Type the ISBN (excluding hyphens) or the title of a book in the Search field to find the page you're looking for.

INTRODUCTION

To the Reader

You might be an absolute beginner with regard to nutrition and physical activity, or you might be a veteran of more weight loss programs than you care to count. Regardless of your experience, this book can help you make sense of the near constant stream of information you get about nutrition, exercise, and your health. Unfortunately, weight loss at any cost seems to be the driving force behind most, if not all, of the health messages we get today. Daily reports on the obesity "epidemic" and its health consequences are enough to make *all* of us—overweight, underweight, and everyone in between—question the status of our physical health. We are inundated with dire statistics about our expanding girths and increased incidence of diseases such as diabetes, cardiovascular disease, and cancer; but these reports do little in the way of actually helping us change our behaviors.

So what's the problem? Why doesn't information do the job? Because today's health messages are based on *avoidance*, and they cannot address the intricacies of behavior change in the real world. In other words, we are taught that we need to quit eating junk food and start exercising, or we face a litany of diseases that, sooner or later, are bound to kill us or destroy our quality of life. We *know* that some foods have little or no nutritional value, but that doesn't change the fact that they are widely available, taste good, and have become stress management tools for many of us! We *know* that exercise is good for our bodies and minds, but too many demands and too little time make regular exercise difficult to accomplish.

Don't get me wrong—avoidance-based information is powerful if you've just suffered a heart attack, been diagnosed with diabetes or cancer, or been lectured by a health care professional about the dangers of your high blood pressure (or if any of the above has happened to a loved one). But if you are fortunate enough to survive, what happens when you are out of immediate danger? Few people are able to maintain motivation to eat well and be physically active when life settles down again. Based on the seriousness of your health issues, you might be able to hold on a little longer than average, but you and I know that ice cream and potato chips still taste as good as they always have.

So what's a health-conscious person to do? Throw caution to the wind? Disregard advice from health professionals? Forget about exercise altogether? Of course not. It's simply time for a fresh approach. Start by letting go of the notion of *perfection* when it comes to health and start thinking about the *process*. Focus on the immediate benefits (like sleeping better, having more energy, or improved interpersonal relationships) instead of dwelling on your risk for disease.

It's my hope that the information in this book differs from typical health information in these three ways:

- It is provided in a positive manner.
- It respects your readiness for lifestyle change.
- It respects you as a person.

You are the only one who knows whether you are ready and able to change your habits. *You* are the only one who can integrate this information into your particular lifestyle. I will provide some guidance with regard to making these decisions, but you have the ultimate responsibility for making it happen. Naturally, then, feel free to pick and choose the changes that make the most sense for you and your current situation. It's impossible to do everything at once, so address your habits one step at a time and be patient with yourself.

One final request—instead of focusing on body weight as the sole or most important measure of success, redirect your efforts toward understanding the *choices and habits* that may influence body weight. Building a healthier lifestyle means reexamining your priorities, rearranging your schedule, and rethinking the way you approach nutrition and fitness. You have a lot of control over your choices, but relatively little control over the number on the scale. For these very reasons, I will forego presenting you with more doom and gloom when it comes to body weight and statistics. You've had enough of that already. I want to address the day-to-day issues, challenges, and potential solutions when it comes to making healthier choices and changing your lifestyle. The information is not new, but I hope you find it presented in a way that is personally meaningful and actionable in your quest for optimal health.

Cheers!

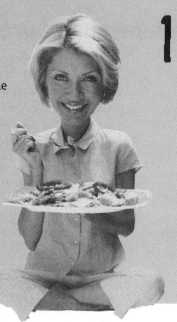

1

Are You Ready?

You are about to begin a lifelong journey toward improved vitality, energy, clarity, and health. In focusing on your health habits, it's critical to understand that these habits fit into a greater whole, which is *you* as a human being. By examining physical health in the context of this greater whole, you will be able to keep the daily ups and downs of changing your habits in their proper place. Changing habits takes time, effort, and commitment, but it should not take over your life. Before you get started, assess your personal "readiness" for this type of commitment and have a realistic picture of your current health.

Dimensions of Wellness

In our quest to achieve "ideal" body weights, we often approach our physical health as though it exists in a vacuum. Nothing could be further from the truth! Physical health is but one of several recognized *dimensions of wellness*. It is certainly the most prominent in our culture, but that fact does not make it any more or less important than the other dimensions. Let's take a moment to put physical health and body weight in the context of the entire *Wellness Wheel*.

The Wellness Wheel (see Figure 1.1) demonstrates how each dimension (physical, occupational, spiritual, social/family, intellectual, and emotional) works together to promote optimal health and quality of life. Each dimension represents the spoke of a bicycle wheel. If all the spokes are functioning properly, the bicycle wheel turns smoothly. However, if one spoke is weak or broken, the wheel is unbalanced and the bicycle is inoperable. This simple concept can be applied to our own personal wellness. If all the dimensions are given appropriate attention, our lives are, to an extent, balanced. On the other hand, if one or more dimensions are ignored or neglected, we cannot reach our full potential in *any* of the areas. Although it is unrealistic to expect to be totally satisfied with every dimension, it makes sense to evaluate where you stand and to act accordingly.

FIGURE 1.1

The Wellness Wheel illustrates the importance of each dimension.

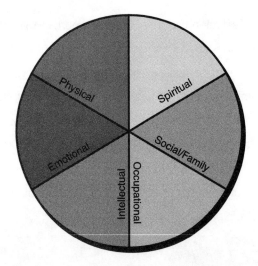

Do imbalances exist in your wellness wheel?

Use Table 1.1 to rate your satisfaction with each dimension of wellness on a scale of 1 to 10, where 1 = very dissatisfied, 5 = somewhat satisfied, and 10 = completely satisfied.

TABLE 1.1   Dimensions of Wellness

Spiritual: 1 2 3 4 5 6 7 8 9 10

6 ■ Your behavior is guided by moral, ethical, and/or religious values.

10 ■ You recognize your purpose in your life; your life has meaning and value.

7 ■ You believe in a higher power, or see yourself as part of a greater whole.

Social/Family: 1 2 3 4 5 6 7 8 9 10

10 ■ You communicate successfully with a wide variety of people.

9 ■ You have developed a network of supportive family members and/or friends.

9 ■ You are able to develop and maintain positive relationships with others.

Intellectual: 1 2 3 4 5 6 7 8 9 10

5 ■ You strive for continued intellectual growth.

5 ■ You deal with new intellectual challenges effectively.

Emotional: 1 2 3 4 5 6 7 8 9 10

2 ■ You express emotions comfortably and appropriately.

2 ■ You manage stress appropriately.

5 ■ You know your own boundaries.

Physical: 1 2 3 4 5 6 7 8 9 10

5 ■ You are free of illness.

3 ■ You are at low risk for medical complications/disease.

2 ■ You have balanced nutrition, exercise, and sleep habits.

Occupational: 1 2 3 4 5 6 7 8 9 10

10 ■ Your organization provides an atmosphere conducive to personal and corporate growth.

9 ■ You have potential for advancement in the company or development within your current position.

9 ■ Your employer is supportive, recognizes accomplishments, and provides feedback.

What are your strongest areas of wellness?

I feel very comfortable with my work and social life, but I think other areas might be suffering.

_____

_____

_____

What are your weakest areas of wellness?

My physical health has been deteriorating because I devote so much time to my job, family, and friends.

_____

_____

_____

What areas are of the greatest value and/or importance to you at this time in your life?

I still value my work and family responsibilities, but I need to find a better balance with physical health now, or I won't be able to be my best self in any area.

_____

_____

_____

Is now the best time for you to focus on the physical dimension of wellness?

Yes, I am ready and willing to commit to changing my habits.

_____

_____

_____

Do other areas require more immediate attention? Which areas? How can you become more satisfied in those areas before attempting to change your nutrition and exercise habits?

No. At this time, physical health is my number one priority. I can always evaluate my overall wellness as I make changes.

_____

_____

_____

These are critical questions to consider. Many people underestimate the amount of time and energy it takes to make lifestyle changes. These changes are positive, but significant stressors, and should be undertaken only after a careful evaluation of your readiness. The following section helps you identify your personal readiness for lifestyle change.

Assessing Your Readiness

Many people jump into exercise and/or dieting with the gusto normally reserved for Olympic competition. Although there are undoubtedly some special cases, most of us would benefit from a more moderate introduction of lifestyle changes. Have you realistically evaluated your current habits? Have you thought about past attempts to eat differently or become more active or both? Now is the time for some personal reflection! The following worksheet is by no means all-inclusive, but it can call attention to important issues when it comes to lifestyle change.

Lifestyle Change: Are You Ready?

Respond with a yes or no to each of the following statements:

1. I understand that changing health habits requires a significant amount of time, energy, and effort.

2. I have evaluated past attempts to change these habits and know what works and what doesn't work for me.

3. I realize that changing health habits can be a significant source of stress, and I am willing to tolerate and manage that stress.

4. I have or am willing to create a "network" of supportive people to help me change my lifestyle.

5. I am willing to try new foods and activities to reach my goals.

6. I am willing to forego immediate weight loss to learn to change my habits for the long haul.

7. I understand that healthy bodies come in many shapes and sizes and that *thin* does not necessarily equal *healthy*, just as *fat* doesn't automatically mean *unhealthy*.

8. I am making these changes for myself, not for someone else or for a special upcoming event.

9. I know that changing my habits is a process, and that I will likely have some setbacks along the way.

10. I rarely eat so much that I feel nauseous, and I do not engage in excessive exercise, purging, or fasting to control my weight.

EVALUATING YOUR RESPONSES

"Yes" responses indicate that you have reasonable expectations and are more likely to be ready to make changes in your eating and activity habits.

"No" responses indicate that you might need to give one or more areas some attention before plunging into lifestyle changes. Read the following explanations to get a better understanding of what to expect and how you might move forward.

The following list provides some direction with respect to each of the statements, which can help you move forward:

1. If the structure or pace of your life at the moment prevents you from devoting extra time and energy to lifestyle change, evaluate whether you can streamline activities or responsibilities. How flexible is your work schedule? Is someone willing to care for your children so you can exercise? Can you delegate responsibilities around the house to free up a little time to plan meals and create grocery lists?

2. Take a long, hard look at previous attempts to change your weight, your habits, or both. Were your expectations realistic? Did you try to do too much, too soon? What were the specific challenges you encountered? Have you resolved some of those challenges, or do you have a different way of handling them?

3. If the thought of adding one more thing to your plate is enough to make you cringe, think twice about jumping into lifestyle change. What are some of the sources of stress in your life? Caring for an aging relative; changing locations, jobs, or careers; a shift in your role in the family; getting married; significant debt; personal illness; pregnancy; strained relationships—all these situations place demands on your entire person. If it's necessary, delay making changes in eating and exercise habits until you get a handle on other important life situations. You are the only person who can determine whether lifestyle change is feasible at this time.

4. If you haven't already, start considering those individuals or groups who can provide the support and encouragement you will need to be successful. (See the section "Your Safety Net: Build Your Support System," in Chapter 2 for more information.)

5. It seems obvious, but if you want to change your health, you're going to have to expand your food and activity horizons. If you're totally averse to experimenting with new foods, ask yourself how you can become a little more adventurous: Choose a new fruit each week, or check out some recipes that look interesting. Expect a little discomfort when increasing your activity level. Discomfort means that you are challenging your body in new ways; pain means you've pushed it too far—understand the difference!

6. Far too many of us seek weight loss at any cost. Trendy diets, excessive exercise, fasting, and dangerous supplements can produce weight loss but don't necessarily improve your health! Changing your daily eating and activity habits, though sometimes arduous and almost always unglamorous, is the only safe, effective method for achieving a healthier body.

7. Each of us was created with a unique genetic code that largely determines our body shape and, to a certain degree, body weight. Have you heard of the "apple" and "pear" shapes in describing bodies? "Apples" tend to store body fat in their stomach, chest, back, and upper body regions, whereas "pears" are more likely to carry fat in their hips, buttocks, and thighs. If you were born an apple, you might become a smaller apple through proper nutrition and exercise, but you will still be an apple! What's more, it's possible to be considered "overweight" by charts and standard definitions but still be in excellent health. Focus on changing behavior instead of changing numbers to keep things in perspective.

8. Lifestyle change comes from the inside out. If you feel pressured into this change, even by a well-meaning friend or loved one, it will not work. Period. Similarly, if your main impetus for change is an upcoming wedding, class reunion, or other special event, it is unlikely you will be able to maintain motivation for the long haul.

9. Lapses are a natural part of the process of change. The successful person takes them for what they are—temporary setbacks that have the potential to be powerful learning tools. Learn to see them as your own personal "scientific experiments." Observe what happened instead of judging it. Evaluate what you can do differently the next time. (More to come in the sections "Managing Lapses" and "Learning from Lapses" in Chapter 2.)

10. These behaviors can indicate serious problems that might require professional attention. Discuss your concerns with a trusted friend, family member, clergy member, therapist, or physician before proceeding.

note

So you're not ready to commit the time and energy it takes to changing health habits? Okay! Take care of higher priority items first, and come back when you're ready, or read the book through and treat it as an exercise in gathering information. This is perfectly acceptable!

Your Current Health Status

Prior to making changes to your eating and activity habits, it is wise to schedule an appointment with your physician for a complete examination. He or she can provide valuable information that will help you tailor a plan specific to your needs. Following your examination, it would also be helpful to schedule an appointment with a certified health and fitness professional at a reputable fitness center to have an individual fitness assessment. This professional can determine your baseline measurements in cardiorespiratory fitness, muscular strength and endurance, flexibility, and body composition. Many people see gains in these areas long before they see changes on the scale; simply knowing that you are making progress can provide needed motivation to stick with new lifestyle habits!

Personal Health Record

Things you need to know and record about yourself before beginning:

- Age (Yes, this is an important one!) _____
- Height (Have I shrunk in the last five years?) _____
- Weight (Not a prerequisite—some people prefer *not* to weigh at all!) _____

WHAT'S A REGISTERED DIETITIAN?

A *registered dietitian (RD)* can be your best ally in making healthier choices about food and eating patterns. Registered dietitians must meet the following criteria to earn and maintain the RD credential:

- Receive a bachelor's degree from an accredited university.
- Complete a supervised practice program.
- Pass a national examination administered by the Commission on Dietetic Registration.
- Complete continuing professional educational requirements to maintain registration.

Find a dietitian in your area at www.eatright.org.

note

Many people claim to be "fitness professionals," but protect yourself by asking about your potential trainer's background. Ideally, he or she should have an undergraduate degree in a health-related background and be certified by a reputable organization such as the American College of Sports Medicine (see www.acsm.org for more details).

note

If you have a personal history of eating disorders, or simply with getting hung up on your body weight, speak with a registered dietitian about whether you should weigh yourself. It's a personal decision, but many people find that focusing on the numbers can actually cause greater harm than good.

Health History

Your health history includes any major surgeries, diagnoses, current or past illness, and so on.

_____

_____

_____

Medications and Supplements

Be sure to tell your physician about any supplements, too.

_____

_____

_____

Weight History

This will help you stay in a relatively realistic frame of mind—see the previous note about whether to weigh yourself.

- Lowest adult weight, maintained ≥ 2 years without formal dieting or excessive exercise _____
- Highest adult weight _____
- Weight range within last five years _____

Blood and Heart Rate Measurements

See Appendix A for more information about desirable levels for these measurements.

- Total blood cholesterol _____mg/dL
- LDL-cholesterol (commonly known as "bad" cholesterol—it's probably not that simple, but it will work for our purposes!) _____mg/dL
- HDL-cholesterol (commonly known as "good" cholesterol) _____mg/dL
- Triglycerides _____mg/dL
- Blood pressure: _____/_____mmHg
- Fasting blood glucose: _____mg/dL (This is important even if you don't have diabetes!)

Other Pertinent Information

_____

_____

_____

The Individual Fitness Assessment

"Why should I put myself through the agony?" you ask. First, you need to know where you are *at this moment in time*. Second, it's cool to see how far you've come after you've implemented some changes. And last, sometimes these are the numbers that can help you stay on track! Contact the American College of Sports Medicine (ACSM) to determine which facilities offer quality assessments by reputable health professionals in your area. ACSM professionals are found around the globe. An individual fitness assessment should include measurements described in each of the following sections.

Cardiorespiratory Fitness

Cardiorespiratory fitness represents the heart's ability to pump blood, the lungs' ability to handle increased volumes of air, and the muscles' ability to utilize oxygen for energy. As your cardiorespiratory fitness improves, your heart becomes more efficient, and you might notice that activities that seemed difficult at first become a little easier. Are you out of breath at the top of the stairs? This is a sign you've challenged your cardiorespiratory system!

Muscular Strength

Strength is the maximum amount of force that can be exerted by a specific muscle or group of muscles. When you heave a large bag of groceries onto the counter, you are displaying muscular strength. Many injuries occur partly because of weakness in either the "working" muscle or its opposing muscle. Incorporating strength training in addition to cardiovascular exercise provides a total approach to fitness.

Chapter 12, "Strength Training 101," introduces you to the benefits and proper methods of strength training, as well as how to develop a training program specific to your fitness level and objectives.

Muscular Endurance

Endurance is the ability of a muscle or group of muscles to contract repeatedly over a period of time long enough to cause fatigue. Muscular endurance is important for posture and performing everyday tasks, such as carrying objects, raking leaves, and leaning, all of which require prolonged muscular exertion.

Flexibility

Flexibility is an indication of your range of motion and an important component of physical fitness. Lack of flexibility in some areas of the body can lead to injury and back pain.

Body Composition

Body composition is simply a measure of how much of your body is lean tissue (bones, muscles, organs, and so forth), and how much is fat tissue. Although our culture seems fixated on body weight as the sole measure of success, body composition may be even more telling. For example, just because a person is at his "ideal" body weight does not automatically mean that he has a healthy level of body fat. And body fat, it seems, is not a static tissue as once believed. Researchers are discovering that our fat tissue sends all kinds of chemical messages to other cells in our bodies, so the amount of fat and that fat's *location* in the body play a pivotal role in our total health profile.

There are many different ways of measuring body composition, some more accurate than others. The gold standard method involves being weighed underwater after you've blown all the air out of your lungs! Sounds fun, doesn't it? Most fitness centers use much more comfortable methods—just be sure that you keep your method consistent when evaluating your progress using body composition. In other words, if you have your body fat measured with skin calipers by a fitness instructor, try to have the same instructor perform the test again six months later when you're ready to see how far you've come.

THE ABSOLUTE MINIMUM

So you think you're ready to go, huh? As you delve into Chapter 2 and beyond, keep these critical points in mind:

- Physical health does not exist in a vacuum.
- Changing health habits is a significant source of stress.
- This may or may not be the appropriate time in your life to address these habits.
- Redefine your definition of success; focus on behaviors rather than numbers.
- A complete physical assessment by your physician and fitness professional provides a great starting point and a standard with which to measure progress.

In This Chapter

- Change is a process with distinct stages
- Build your support system or risk failure
- Keep records to ensure success
- Develop smart goals
- Learn from your mistakes

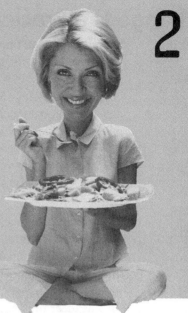

2

The Stages Of Change— What To Expect

Perhaps you are not actually an absolute beginner at trying to change your health habits. (And who is in this age of "health as religion"!?) You may be a veteran dieter or a weekend warrior who has gained and lost the same 10, 20, 50, or 100 pounds or more, many times over. You might think you have a willpower "problem." You might feel overwhelmed by the magnitude of the changes you want to make. Illness or vacation might have thrown you far from the nutrition and exercise bandwagon in the past. If you find yourself nodding in agreement with any or all of these statements, it's time to *stop* participating in self-defeating attitudes and habits, *look* at the alternatives available in your unique situation, and *listen* to what your own body is telling you.

Change Is a Process

Before you can accomplish those three things, however, you must have a firm understanding of the framework for behavior change. Change is a *process* with distinct stages through which you must progress to realize your ultimate goal. Find comfort in knowing that you might not necessarily work through these stages in the exact order in which they are presented, and you may go back and forth between several stages before progressing. In this chapter, you'll find concrete tools and techniques that can facilitate movement from one stage to the next, so take it one step at a time and go at your own pace! Refer to this chapter as you work your way through the rest of the book. It will help you stay focused and keep things in perspective.

The Stages of Change (see Figure 2.1), first conceptualized by psychologists James Prochaska and Carlo DiClemente in the late 1970s and early 1980s, can be applied to any type of behavior modification, including diet, exercise, smoking cessation, or implementing any new habit. The following information should help you get a better understanding of characteristics shared by individuals in each of the stages and provide ideas that empower you to move forward.

FIGURE 2.1

The Stages of Change illustrate that change is a *process*, not an *event*.

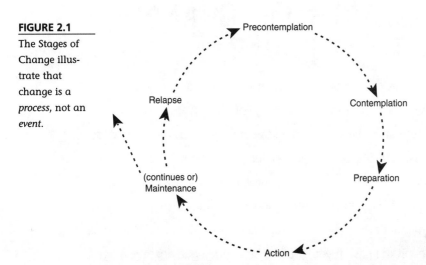

Precontemplation: Who, Me? Change? No Way!

People in the first stage of change typically

- Have no interest in making a behavior change
- Might not be aware a change needs to be made

- Do not intend, or are not ready, to change
- Deny that a problem exists
- Might have previously attempted to change the target behavior and "failed"

With regard to nutrition and physical activity, it is unlikely you are still in this stage. You've read this far, right? If you know someone in precontemplation, the most important thing you can provide him is empathy. Ask her how she feels about the target behavior, and truly listen to the answer. Invite him to a seminar or class he may find enjoyable. Nagging, though common, is *not* the best method for helping a person move beyond this stage! If you feel you must take some kind of action, you might leave magazine articles or informational brochures in conspicuous places as a nonthreatening way of broaching the subject. Sometimes the hardest step is letting your loved ones come to a stage of readiness on their own instead of pushing them toward change.

Contemplation: Maybe I Should Think About It...

People in the second stage of change typically

- Think about changing
- Consider ways to make the change
- Know a change would be good, but don't feel ready or able to change right now
- Do not plan to change within one month

You may identify closely with contemplation at this time. Some people linger in this stage for years, waiting for the right time to begin the process. You think, "after I get through this busy time at work," or "I'll just follow this diet to lose weight for (fill in the blank: wedding, class reunion, interview, and so on), and then learn how to eat more healthfully," or "when the kids don't require so much from me at home..." Guess what? There is no perfect time to begin the process! Certainly, it is wise to take care of overwhelming or chaotic situations first (that's why you went to the trouble of assessing your readiness in Chapter 1, "Are You Ready?"), but life is probably always going to be full. The bottom line is this—we all have 24 hours a day, and making health a *priority* is going to make the difference.

At this point, try to connect with people who have already made a change similar to the one you are considering. Talk to them; learn more about their methods, setbacks, and successes. Become aware of alternatives in your own environment. Join a support group.

Seek an exercise environment that appeals to *you*. Visit fitness centers in your area to get a feel for the atmosphere and philosophy of each. Many fitness centers have temporary or trial memberships so that you can experience them yourself. If the thought of spandex and exposed flesh gives you nightmares, and you can't find a "friendly" gym in your area, create your own home fitness center with simple hand weights, a jump rope, some stairs or any other innovative "equipment" you can find! Brush the cobwebs off your old clunker bike in the garage. Look for walking or biking paths in your city. An aversion to using fancy equipment is *not* an excuse to be a couch potato! Chapter 13, "Exercising at Home and on the Road," provides guidance for creating a fit environment no matter your location.

note

If you struggle with overeating, *Overeaters Anonymous* is a worldwide support network with a philosophy based on the familiar 12-step programs. Find a location near you at www.overeatersanonymous.org, or contact your local chapter.

Preparation: I Think I Can, I Think I Can...

People in the third stage of change typically

- Acknowledge that the pros of change outweigh the cons of not changing
- Intend to make a change within one month
- May be making small changes already

Many of you are currently in the preparation stage, so I'm going to devote a little extra space to some tools you can use to take it to the next level. At this point, you have already made the decision to change; it is now imperative to have a support system of trustworthy friends, relatives, co-workers, and health professionals to help you advance from preparation to action. Stick with one or two small changes at a time, allow those to become habit, and then move on to new or more challenging areas.

tip

If you're thinking, "I hate to exercise, I always have, and I always will," now's the time to rethink your definition of success when it comes to getting active. Start by simply moving more. You've heard it already—park farther from the entrance of the building; take the stairs instead of the elevator; walk on your lunch break. These activities might not qualify as exercise, but they most certainly require energy and can produce health benefits. Start with simple ways to increase your daily movement and worry about the "exercise stuff" later.

Your Safety Net: Build Your Support System

The importance of developing a strong network of support in achieving healthier habits cannot be overstated! This is not the time to be an island. Think about individuals who can provide support, encouragement, and guidance on your path to improved physical health. Nothing is more discouraging than feeling like you are swimming against a tide of resistance to healthy behaviors in your home, work, or other environment. And the fact of the matter is that the people surrounding us on a daily basis can influence our health behaviors in both positive and negative ways.

Have you ever tried to order a soup and salad while your dinner companions are pushing the Mega-Burger and home fries? What about the relative who consistently places seconds and thirds on your plate after you've politely refused? Has a loved one ever openly chastised you for having dessert or commented on your weight gain? Try going for an afternoon walk when your supervisor scrutinizes every move you make. These individuals, though usually well meaning, often present some of the greatest challenges you will face in changing your habits.

On the other hand, the people we choose to keep in our inner circles can also be powerful motivators for *positive* behavior change. Try to appoint several "key figures" for your support network—a family member, a friend, a co-worker, a spiritual advisor, and a health professional—to help you stay on track. Ask these people whether they would be willing to be your *accountability partners* in weight management. They are not responsible for your decisions, but they are willing to be your cheerleaders, exercise partners, advisors, and counselors. They may or may not be trying to make similar changes.

For example, even though your best friend of 20 years may never struggle with his weight, he could be a perfect walking or running partner. A co-worker who mentioned that she is trying to eat more healthfully would make an excellent lunch date. A registered dietitian can help you devise a sensible meal plan that works for your particular lifestyle. The most important thing is to *tell* these people what you are trying to accomplish and *ask* whether they'd be willing to help.

caution

Sometimes, the people closest to you may *not* make the best accountability partners for your particular needs. They may have a difficult time being objective because they are so closely involved in your life; they may fear that the change you want to make will have a direct effect on their lifestyle (it probably will to some extent); and frankly, change can be frightening, especially when it's taking place in someone near and dear to you. This doesn't mean they can't help; it just means that you may need to rely more heavily on other individuals for support in certain areas. You are the only one who can make this determination—choose wisely!

Key to Success: Keep Records

Beyond your support network, you'll need to start holding *yourself* accountable for your behaviors. One of the most reliable predictors of success in lifestyle management is *self-monitoring*. Self-monitoring by keeping accurate records of your actions and attitudes can be as simple or as complex as you care—the important thing is to be consistent. By recording this information, you gain self-direction, motivation, accountability, and a means of monitoring progress. The following is a laundry list of everything you could potentially record, but don't feel obligated to go into this much detail. I have many clients who scribble their food and activity choices in a little pocket notebook, and that works just as well. See Figure 2.2 for a sample food log.

- Your food choices:
    - What you eat
    - How much you eat
    - When you eat
    - Your eating location/environment
    - Your level of hunger and fullness before and after eating (more to come in Chapter 3, "Uncover the Natural Eater"!)
    - Your emotions, feelings, and/or thoughts before, during, and after eating
- Your activity choices:
    - What type
    - How long
    - What time of day
    - Level of difficulty (on a scale of 0 to 10; see the section "Rating of Perceived Exertion" in Chapter 11 for more details)
    - Your heart rate
    - Your emotions, feelings, and/or thoughts before, during, and after the activity
- Your personal goals:
    - Personal motivations
    - Long-term goals
    - Short-term goals
    - Daily steps to success

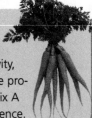

note

Blank food, activity, and goal logs are provided in Appendix A for your convenience.

FIGURE 2.2

Your food logs should look something like this sample.

Daily Food Choices

Date:_____   Day of week:_____

Time	Hunger/Fullness Rating Pre-Meal/Post-Meal	Amount	Food or Beverage	Location	Feelings
7:00 am	Pre 3 / Post 6	8 oz 2 cups 1 slice 2 tsp 8 oz 8 oz	2% milk Frosted Flakes cereal wheat toast butter orange juice coffee with cream and sugar	Kitchen counter	rushed
10:00 am	Pre 2 / Post 4	1 medium	glazed donut	break room	guilty; starving

Goals:

Challenges:

Smart Goals

One of the most common mistakes people make when changing health habits is setting only a *weight* goal. There are several reasons why goal weights can be self-defeating:

- **Numbers never tell the entire story.** You know those annoying height and weight charts, or the newer body mass index tables? Talk about feeling like a lost cause! Some of you may never fit neatly into the charts and tables. Does that mean you can't be healthy? Not necessarily! Most research shows that it's better to be "overweight" and *active* than at your "ideal weight" (if such a thing exists) and *inactive*. Another caveat of using the scale to measure success is that body *weight* doesn't correlate well with body *composition*. In other words, you can be a slender person who carries a lot of body fat, or a heavy person who carries a lot of muscle tissue. That's why we emphasized having your body composition measured in Chapter 1, "Are You Ready?"

- **Body weight fluctuates on a daily basis.** Changes in body weight over the course of a day or two reflect nothing more than water balance. If you've eaten a salty meal or snack (remember the pretzels you had yesterday afternoon and the tasty little grains of salt you licked from the bottom of the bag?), you might be retaining fluid and weigh a couple pounds heavier than normal. If, on the other hand, you decide to hop on the scale after a brisk walk or jog in hot, humid weather, you're likely to be dehydrated and weigh a pound or two less than normal. Does this mean you burned two pounds of fat in the last hour? Unfortunately, this isn't the case. You've lost some water through sweat and evaporation, and it's time to drink up! More specifically, you'll need to drink 16 ounces of fluid (about .5 liters) for every pound of body weight lost during exercise (this guideline is accurate only if weighing "conditions" are similar before and after exercise—in the buff is best!) Women also experience fluctuations in body weight throughout the menstrual cycle, mostly due to fluid retention.

> **tip**
>
> Hydration status has been the subject of much debate in recent years. Chapter 4, "Balanced Nutrition," contains a more complete explanation of the importance of getting the right amount of fluids for your particular needs. For now, it's a good bet to take this simple test—observe the color and frequency of your urine. If you relieve yourself every few hours (or more frequently), and your urine is fairly pale, you're getting enough fluid. If not, bottom's up!

- **Weighing can be very emotionally charged.** If you weigh yourself on a regular basis without feeling guilty or righteous after seeing the number on the scale, more power to you. For most of us, that's probably not the case. If you've ever starved yourself before going to the doctor's office (or any other "official" weigh in), or feasted afterward, it's probably best if you weigh yourself as little as possible. It's too easy to let a number sabotage your best efforts. The fit of your clothes or even your undergarments can serve the very same purpose without carrying the same emotional "weight" as the number on the scale.

- **If weight loss is your only motivation, what happens when you reach your goal?** Many "successful" dieters can't stay motivated when they aren't experiencing the excitement of weight loss—the compliments, the new clothes, or the drama of seeing an old friend in their new body. Don't become a dieting casualty. You are in this for the long haul, and chances are good that your weight is going to fluctuate given your life circumstances. Focus on the things that matter, such as feeding yourself well, walking whenever you can, and balancing your physical health with other priorities!

Have I convinced you *not* to make body weight *per se* a goal? I hope so! But the question remains: How do you formulate positive, effective, action-oriented personal goals? In general, you'll want to follow the simple progression illustrated in Figure 2.3.

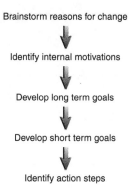

FIGURE 2.3

Develop smart goals with a logical progression.

Begin by listing some of the reasons for changing your habits in Figure 2.4. List as many as you can. Try for more than 25! In general, the most powerful personal motivations will emerge at end of your list. You may begin by listing "fit into my clothes better" or "have more energy" and work your way down to "improve my relationship with my spouse/children/grandchildren" or "get the confidence I need to change careers." Now you're talking! These internal motivations for change will provide the foundation you need to set concrete long- and short-term goals and begin to take action on a daily basis.

After you identify your key internal motivations, honestly evaluate what it will take to get you there. This process will allow you to develop simple, effective long- and short-term goals, as well as pinpoint the action steps necessary to meet those goals. Let's take a look at how this process might play out:

> Cindy was getting ready to retire. She and her husband had raised three children and were looking forward to traveling, relaxing, and spending more time with their family. In taking care of her family's needs before her own, Cindy had reached a point where she didn't like how she looked, felt, or moved. After spending a little time brainstorming all the potential reasons for changing her habits, she determined that her deepest desire and greatest motivation was to improve her confidence level. She had been active throughout her childhood, adolescence, and young adulthood and knew how much better she felt at those times in her life; therefore, one of her long-term goals was to become a regular exerciser. It had been at least 20 years since she had been regularly active, so she knew she needed to start modestly. Her first short-term goal was to walk for 15 minutes before work on Monday, Wednesday, and Friday. Cindy decided on the following action steps, each to be done in the evenings: Lay out walking clothes and shoes, pack a lunch for the following day, and then set the alarm clock 20 minutes earlier than usual.

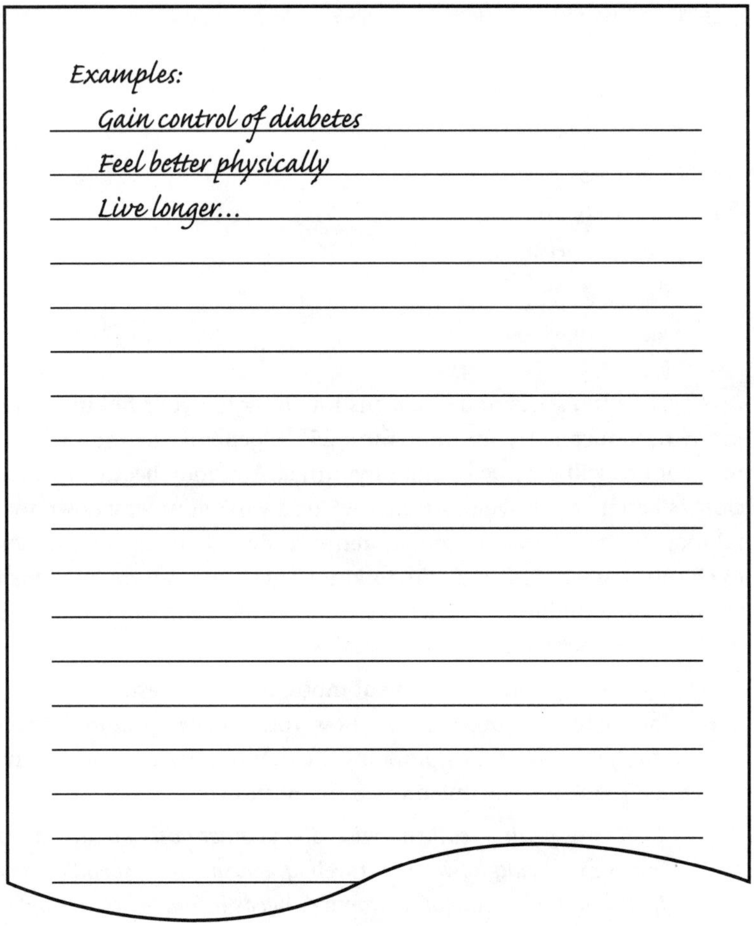

FIGURE 2.4
Reasons to change my habits. (We'll get you started.)

Examples:

Gain control of diabetes

Feel better physically

Live longer...

Now it's your turn! Look over your reasons for change and identify common values and themes. These are your internal motivations—the deep-seated beliefs and desires that will form the foundation of your plan to change.

What are your personal motivations?

_____

_____

_____

What will it take to get you there?

_____

_____

_____

Identify your top two long-term goals that reflect your internal motivations.

1. _____

_____

2. _____

_____

Now break them down into more manageable steps. These are your short-term goals.

    1. _____

        a. _____

        b. _____

    2. _____

        a. _____

        b. _____

        c. _____

Finally, choose one or more short-term goals on which to focus and list the action steps you can take *this week* to meet those goals.

This week, I will _____

_____

_____

Write down your goals and keep them visible. Post them on the bathroom mirror, the refrigerator, or your computer's monitor. By focusing on positive steps, you can begin to develop a mindset that will ensure success. Remember the acronym *BE SMART* when formulating your personal goals, especially in the short term:

    Behavior-oriented

    Expectations, be realistic

    Specific details

    Measurable objectives

    Attainability

    Rewards put into place

    Time frame identified

Identifying the *behavior* you want to change and habits that feed the desired behavior is essential in goal setting. Be *realistic* with your *expectations*. If it took 10 years to gain 20 pounds, don't expect to lose the excess weight in a few months. Allow yourself to succeed at small steps by identifying *specific, measurable, and attainable objectives.* (For example, "I will drink water instead of soda for lunch at least three days this week" instead of "I will drink more water.") Give yourself an incremental *reward system* for achieving your goals. A night at the movies, a new exercise video, a relaxing bath, or a golf outing for short-term goals; plan a vacation, buy a new suit, throw a celebration, for example, as rewards for achieving long-term goals. Remember to set a specific *time frame* for a goal, such as two weeks or a month, so that you will have some basis for rewarding your achievements. If you haven't met your goal by the specified time, simply reevaluate the situation. Do you need to approach it from a different angle with new action steps? Perhaps you want to change the nature of the goal altogether. Either way, by setting the time frame, you will make progress consistently rather than erratically.

Action: Just Do It!

People in the fourth stage of change typically

- Have been practicing new behavior for less than six months
- Feel in control and empowered much of the time
- Are at the greatest risk for lapse and relapse

Congratulations, you are doing it! (Well, maybe not quite yet, but you will be!) This is the most visible stage in the entire process. Friends and family members may be asking about your new behaviors; you may be getting compliments about your appearance or energy level. Enjoy it! However, be aware that temptations are going to hit you like freight trains, and it's up to you to treat setbacks, or lapses, as learning experiences rather than failures. Now is the time to be patient and to critically and objectively examine any lapses in behavior to develop strategies that meet challenges in a more appropriate fashion.

Managing Lapses

Lapses occur in almost every person's journey to a healthier lifestyle. We all have ways of coping with life's challenges, but our methods aren't always conducive to physical health. From food binges to long periods without physical activity, lapses have

> **note**
>
> A *relapse* essentially means that you have regressed to an earlier stage (often precontemplation or contemplation) in the Stages of Change. It's not the end of the world; it simply means you need time for some personal reflection before you are ready to try again. If this happens to you, start from the beginning and reassess your readiness for lifestyle change.

been the downfall of many a New Year's resolution. How can you prevent a lapse in healthy behavior from progressing to an all out *relapse*?

The key is a new approach to everyday challenges. If and when a lapse occurs, seize the opportunity to examine the situation and develop a specific intervention for the next time the same situation arises. See Table 2.1 for some examples of common high-risk situations and their potential interventions. There is no one "correct" way to prevent unwanted behaviors from recurring. The best intervention is one that fits your needs, lifestyle, and personality!

Table 2.1 Common High-Risk Situations and Potential Interventions

Situation	Intervention
I wasn't that hungry when my kids were eating lunch, so I just skipped it. Later that afternoon, I was ravenous and found myself eating whatever wasn't nailed to the floor.	You can't always wait for the perfect time to eat. Sometimes, it makes sense to eat at least a small snack to prevent a "crisis" situation from occurring in a few hours. Have some fruit and roasted nuts at lunch time if you're just slightly hungry.
I always get hungry at work before lunch and find myself gravitating towards the only food in my building: the vending machines.	At the beginning of the week, prepare snack bags of nutritious foods such as carrots, string cheese, and small containers of peanuts or almonds to leave at work. Bring a bag of mixed fresh fruit to keep on your desk or in the office refrigerator. When you get the midmorning munchies, you will be armed with a healthy alternative.
I have a habit of automatically eating when I sit down to watch television at night.	Instead of letting your television viewing area be a place for eating, make it a no-food zone. If necessary, turn off the TV for a full week to break the cycle. Most people are amazed at the time (and calories!) they spend in front of the television.
I went on vacation last month, my clothes don't fit, and I haven't been able to get back to my walking program since. Ack!	Vacations and breaks from your normal routine are a vital part of maintaining your enthusiasm for life in general. Right now, lace up your shoes, grab your dog or any willing companion, and head outside. Commit to walking for five minutes. When you're finished, you have the option of coming back inside (but I bet you'll want to keep going!). Sometimes, the law of inertia is your worst enemy. The next time you go on vacation, try to plan a little activity into your itinerary. Can you go camping? Schedule a walking or biking tour of your destination? Get up a little early to catch a gorgeous sunrise and stretch your legs a bit? It's easier to get back into your routine at home if you've maintained even a minimal level of activity while you were away. Chapter 13 is chock full of tips and ideas to help you accomplish this in a sane and convenient fashion.

What are some of *your* high-risk situations? Can you think of an intervention for each? Create your own list of situations and how you plan to react to them positively.

Learning from Lapses

Keep a log of your lapse experiences. Find patterns in your behavior so that you can modify your environment and plan ahead for the next time you are faced with a similar situation:

- What were you feeling?
- Where were you?
- With whom were you keeping company?
- What was the time of day?

It also might be helpful to jot down a *behavior chain* in a journal. This involves nothing more than writing down the series of events, situations, feelings, emotions, or experiences that led to the unwanted behavior. Your behavior chain might look something like this:

- I was having a decent day at work.
- My supervisor asked whether she could speak with me in her office.
- She proceeded to tell me that our department would have to make some changes and that my colleague and good friend would be leaving.
- It would be my responsibility to perform his job duties until we could find a more suitable arrangement.
- I was overwhelmed and angry.
- I drove home in a "stew."
- When I got inside, I went directly to the kitchen to decide what to have for dinner.
- Nothing looked good.
- A package of cookies was on the counter, so I ate a few of those while I pondered what to fix.

note

Many people who have just experienced a lapse remark, "I don't know what happened. Before I knew it, I was just (you fill it in: eating an entire box of cookies, skipping my workouts, ordering a mighty mocha triple fudge coffee beverage at the local cafe, and so on)." Let's face it, behaviors don't just "happen." On some level, you chose to partake in those activities because they offered something you needed: pleasure, a release, relaxation, or more time for other responsibilities. The key behavior that separates successful from unsuccessful people is a willingness to figure out just what those true needs are and seek new ways of meeting them.

- Still couldn't find anything that looked good, so I had some chips, too.

- Settled on a frozen pizza but was really hungry, so I took the bag of chips into the living room and turned on the TV while I waited for the pizza to bake.

- When it was done, I was already engrossed in the TV program, so I took the pizza into the living room, too.

- By the end of the show, I had eaten six slices of pizza and felt sick to my stomach; I was too tired to go for a walk.

- I cleaned up and berated myself for being such a glutton; then resolved to "do better" the next day.

Sound familiar? I'm sure you could share countless similar stories. Why go through the agony of writing it down? Because seeing it on paper demystifies the unwanted behavior. It's easy to understand why you ate six slices of pizza when you take the day's events into consideration. If you can get a handle on the purpose your behavior was serving, you can identify alternatives that meet the real need. Seek the help of a counselor, minister, or therapist if you need help identifying or determining how best to meet these needs.

tip

The earlier you can break your behavior chain, the better! For example, if something stressful happens at work, don't wait until you're standing in front of the refrigerator to take action. Go for a walk that afternoon to give yourself a chance to mull it over. When you get home, do something that gives you a sense of control— wash your car, clean a drawer, or go for a run. Do whatever it takes to break the cycle!

Maintenance: A Habit Is Formed

Let's bring it back to our Stages of Change now for the grand finale. People in the fifth stage of change typically

- Have been practicing new behaviors for six months or more

- Consider the new behavior part of their lifestyle

- View lapses as temporary setbacks and know how to implement coping strategies

At this point, healthy behaviors have become a part of your lifestyle. In this stage, boredom and complacency may be your worst enemies. Try new approaches to help maintain your healthy habits: Participate in a group fitness class, choose a new food or recipe each month, or expand your cultural horizons by attending a play or an art show. Continue to talk to others about the changes you have made. Start a support group; schedule a follow-up fitness assessment; meet with a registered dietitian; enjoy your new, healthier body!

Accountability and Perspective (Willis's Story)

Willis (not his real name) says that he has had a weight challenge for most of his life. As a young man in the armed services, he was able to maintain a normal weight through required, rigorous physical activity, but after retiring, he struggled in the absence of that accountability. With a strong family history of Type 2 Diabetes, he knew that he couldn't continue to gain weight and remain inactive without suffering consequences.

"My sister's passing at the age of 66 due to complications from diabetes was a real wake-up call. I knew I needed to get serious about eating right and exercising, so I started walking—not fast—and eating less food. I lost an average of 2 pounds a week for 52 weeks—not nearly as fast as most people expect to lose, but I was consistent."

Willis credits his success to accountability and long-range perspective.

"Everyone needs accountability in some form. For me, it was joining NIFS (the National Institute for Fitness and Sport) and setting a schedule. Other people need accountability outside of themselves. You also have to understand that lifestyle change is a process, not an event. You need to look long range. Think about being there for your grandchildren, enjoying your retirement years, things like that. You need to be able to *engage* in life."

Willis readily admits that it isn't always easy and that he continues to educate himself as much as possible about nutrition and health-related topics. His advice for people who find it difficult to recover from lapses and setbacks is to establish more accountability. He did this for himself by becoming a small group leader in the NIFS Mini Marathon training program.

"Get in a structured exercise program, and beyond that, put yourself in a leadership position within that program. Be willing to commit yourself and care enough to lead others. For me, that made all the difference."

When asked about maintaining motivation after you've had some initial success, Willis responds, "That's when the long-range perspective becomes so important."

A lot of people do this to look good, and some people do this to be able to participate in activities of life, and some people exercise to keep their organs healthy. I think there's a place for all three. Develop goals that meet all three—and know that you don't need to make these changes instantly."

THE ABSOLUTE MINIMUM

Do you have a feel for your current position within the Stages of Change? If not, look back through the descriptions of individuals in each stage. You need to understand where you are now so that you'll be able to navigate the uncharted territory of new behaviors.

- Change is a process that happens in the minutia of everyday living—small steps count.

- Support is essential—find it in as many places as possible.

- Set goals that are smart, are action-oriented, and reflect your personal beliefs, values, and attitudes.

- Start recording your behaviors in whatever way you feel most comfortable—perhaps a journal, or refer to Appendix A, "Worksheets and Additional Resources" for sample food, activity, and goal logs.

- Treat yourself with the same consideration you might show a good friend; when you make a mistake, evaluate what happened, plan what to do the next time, and move on!

IN THIS CHAPTER

- Why diets are recipes for disaster
- Understand your personal eating pattern
- Learn to identify and respond to your body's natural signals
- Become a mindful eater

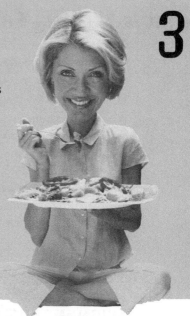

3

UNCOVER THE NATURAL EATER

Have you ever observed a toddler's eating behavior? Young children generally practice *natural eating* at its best. There are exceptions to every rule, but most children exposed to a wide variety of nutritious foods will balance calorie and nutrient intake over the course of several days or weeks to meet their needs for normal growth and development. When they're hungry, they are interested only in finding the next meal or snack; when their tummies are full, they cannot be coerced into taking another bite! Granted, toddlers have many advantages over adults in this regard—their schedules are flexible, their stress levels are low, and media influence and exposure to advertisements don't exert quite as much power—but the busy, health-conscious adult can learn a lot from their style of eating. This chapter is devoted to helping you uncover your own natural eater.

What *Is* Natural Eating?

Do you remember a time in your life when food was simply food? You ate when you were hungry, stopped when you were satisfied, and beyond food preparation and cleanup (if you were old enough), you spent relatively little time thinking about it. That is natural eating.

What if you cannot remember *ever* feeling this way about food? Perhaps for as long as you have known, food has been associated with everything *but* the messages your own body was sending. You might have been raised in an environment that did not support natural eating, one in which your access to food was overly restricted or you were required to ignore your body's hunger or fullness signals. Or you may have fallen victim to the dieting culture so prevalent today, the one that promises that happiness is just a few more pounds away. If this is the case, don't despair. As a human being, you were born with the ability to regulate food intake appropriately, and you can begin to uncover this ability again by working through some of the steps in the following sections.

NATURAL EATING OCCURS INDEPENDENTLY OF BODY WEIGHT

Becoming a natural eater is not a guarantee that you will change your body weight. People who maintain unnaturally thin physiques will probably gain weight as they begin to respect their bodies again. People who are maintaining excess weight due to environmental, emotional, or other conditions will probably lose weight as they incorporate the principles of natural eating. If you have ignored your body's signals for a long time by chronically over- or undereating (or going back and forth between the two), it may be more challenging to decipher appropriate hunger and fullness signals. If you believe you may be such a person, work with your physician, a counselor, and a registered dietitian to develop an eating plan and healthy lifestyle that respects this history.

The vast majority of people can experience the freedom of becoming a natural eater by working through the material in this book and using other appropriate resources. Know that it may be a long and sometimes uncomfortable process, but the reward of a peaceful relationship with food and your body is worth every bit of effort you can afford!

For more information on this subject, consider reading *Intuitive Eating: a Revolutionary Program That Works* by Evelyn Tribole and Elyse Resch (St. Martins, 2003).

Before we get into the specifics of natural eating, let's talk about what it *isn't*.

Natural Eating Is *Not* a Diet

The end goal of every diet is weight loss, and in theory weight loss is simple—you have to consistently burn more calories (energy) than you consume. Unfortunately, this "simple" matter of energy balance is difficult to navigate behaviorally. Genetics, culture, social habits, motivation, and countless other factors affect whether you can lose weight and maintain the loss. Many individuals diet without considering the harm they may be inflicting on their bodies and minds or what is actually required to maintain a healthy weight for the rest of their lives. If you have been on and off diets for as long as you can remember or are considering a diet now, know this—you do not fail on a diet; the dieting process fails *you*.

Why Do Diets Fail You?

Diets are destined to fail you because

- Diets do not address all the factors related to food choices.
- Diets focus on the scale instead of behavior changes.
- Diets do not often include, encourage, or promote physical activity.
- Diets do not require a lifestyle change.
- Diets have a beginning and an end.
- Diets create a parent/child relationship with food (being "good" or "bad" when you eat, or avoid, certain foods) that frequently leads to rebellious eating.
- Diets do not require you to change the way you think about food.
- Your body desires weight stability and will go to great lengths to maintain your current weight.

What Does Work?

To succeed at changing your health habits, you must be willing to learn new attitudes and behaviors related to nutrition, physical activity, and life balance. It is absolutely critical to examine your current lifestyle to determine which factors are perpetuating unhealthy behaviors. It may be

- A sedentary work environment
- A lack of social support
- Increased reliance on convenience foods
- Unmanaged stress

Some individuals can quickly adopt new behaviors; others have deep-seated emotional and/or psychological barriers to eating healthfully or being active. You must examine these barriers, preferably with the help of a counselor or therapist, prior to or in conjunction with learning new behaviors, even if that interferes with immediate change. In the end, a healthy person is one who learns to enjoy all foods in moderation, consistently engages in physical activity, and copes with life challenges in an appropriate fashion.

Take a moment now for some personal reflection. Putting your ideas in writing in Figure 3.1 will help you get a handle on some of the challenges in your own life and can prevent you from wasting time and energy fighting an enemy you can't see.

FIGURE 3.1

My personal healthy habit challenges.

Some of the issues/challenges I expect to face while working toward a healthier lifestyle include

EXAMPLE:

I have young children at home and time is a huge issue in planning, shopping for, and preparing healthy meals.

Two small steps I can take to begin managing these challenges are

1. *I can ask if other parents in my community would be open to arranging "kid swaps" so that we all have time to do groceries and run errands.*

2. *I can borrow quick and healthy cookbooks from the public library to get ideas for simple, family-friendly meals.*

3.

4.

What Is a Healthy Weight?

Although this is a book designed to help you improve your habits, many of you are also curious about what constitutes a healthy body weight. First and foremost, it's important to remember that weight is simply a number. As you learned in Chapter 2, "The Stages of Change—What to Expect," focusing on body weight as a goal can be counterproductive for a number of reasons, but because we live in a weight-obsessed age, this topic merits further discussion.

For many individuals, a modest loss of even 5% of current body weight can improve health parameters such as blood pressure, blood sugar, and blood cholesterol levels. Unfortunately, most people who embark on weight loss programs begin with completely unrealistic goals—they report an inability to be satisfied with modest, but beneficial weight loss. This kind of all-or-nothing mentality is a recipe for frustration, body dissatisfaction, and preoccupation with body weight and appearance. For these reasons, I will not use typical methods employed by many organizations and professionals to determine your "ideal" body weight (there's nothing inherently wrong with the charts and tables; it's simply more productive to focus your energy elsewhere). If you prefer, go back to the section on your personal weight history and use this information as a starting point to determine a healthy weight *range*. Choose a range that you were able to maintain as an adult without dieting or excessive exercise but that reflects adequate nutrition, regular activity, and attention to overall health.

Another important consideration is respect for your basic body type. Many people attempt to change their body shapes with dieting and exercising only to become frustrated, tired, and obsessed with their various imperfections. It's an unfortunate result of a culture that has little regard for the beauty of genetic diversity in body types or the inherent worth of a person's soul and character. Learn to work with the wonderful body you've been given. You don't have to be enamored with every last inch, but do try to see yourself in a positive light.

In the same way that your genes determine where you store body fat, they will determine how you lose that fat. Do you have illusions of reducing body fat in select areas of your body? Many women, for example, are frustrated by the apparent tenacity of fat stores in their hips and thighs (or other areas of the body). Although balanced nutrition and regular exercise can improve many health parameters and decrease *overall* body fat, women must accept the fact that they are biologically wired to store fat in these areas. Keep this in mind if you are embarking on a weight loss program with someone of the opposite gender!

Again, focus on changing behaviors, and you will naturally arrive at a healthier weight. Identifying your eating style or styles is an important first step in changing your eating behaviors and working toward becoming a natural eater.

Evaluate Your Current Eating Pattern

To identify your eating pattern, you must be willing to evaluate your relationship with food and eating. Humans have all sorts of reasons for eating—celebration, stress, boredom, comfort, loneliness, pleasure, social situations, cultural traditions, control, anxiety, habit, and countless others that have little or nothing to do with a physiological need for nourishment. The beauty of natural eating lies in its ability to both fulfill your body's need for energy and respect your unique mind, heart, and soul. Does this mean that you should never eat for purely social, cultural, or emotional reasons? Absolutely not. By becoming a natural eater, you'll begin to understand how your body adjusts for these situations and provides you with reliable hunger and fullness signals to reestablish your connection with eating's original purposes.

Sound like a bunch of feel-good jargon? I will identify several eating patterns so that you can relate to these concepts on a more personal level. I've included examples of life situations that illustrate each pattern, but you may exhibit characteristics of the pattern without matching any of the examples. You'll also find that you probably fall into more than one category depending on the situation at hand. The label isn't as important as your willingness to examine all the ways in which you might use food.

Restrained Eating

The *restrained eater* often appears to be the picture of health. He may work out religiously, scrutinize his food choices, and keep close tabs on his body weight. Below the surface, however, the restrained eater agonizes over food choices and may miss out on social events due to erratic eating and exercise patterns. He spends an inordinate amount of time thinking about food, planning what to eat or avoid, and/or exercising to "make up" for indulgences. The restrained eater may look like the textbook definition of health, but he is far from achieving a balanced lifestyle or peace of mind. Many dieters fall into this category when they religiously count calories, points, or grams of carbohydrate, fat, or protein. For some restrained eaters, food is the one thing over which they exert full control, so eating becomes their method of coping with an otherwise unpredictable life.

Chaotic Eating

The *chaotic eater* runs at full throttle day in and day out. She may juggle a full-time job with family and community responsibilities and often works long hours, stealing time from exercise and/or sleep to please as many people as possible. The chaotic eater frequently uses convenience foods and rarely sits down at a table to eat. She might eat in the car, on the bus, at her desk, during meetings, or while talking on the phone or answering emails. Her life is fast, and so is her food. She knows she should feed herself more nutritiously, but life is simply too hectic to make it a top priority.

Chaotic eaters spend a lot of time at the extremes of hunger and fullness. They may go many hours or most of the day with nothing more than coffee and a vending machine snack, and then gorge themselves at night when they finally have the opportunity. Other chaotic eaters simply don't want to be bothered with planning nutritious meals and snacks. They believe that tedious task is reserved for health nuts and nutrition professionals. Dieting veterans can be chaotic eaters when they are "off" their diets; they reason that they'll get back on the bandwagon when life slows down a bit and they can muster a little more willpower.

> **note**
>
> Willpower is *not* the most reliable ally when it comes to changing your lifestyle. It's the first thing to go when you're tired, hungry, stressed, or bored. Instead of trying to change your reaction to the environment (willpower), figure out how to change the environment itself. *(stress)*

Emotional Eating

The *emotional eater* turns to food to lessen the intensity of negative emotions and enhance the enjoyment of positive emotions. He is usually sensitive to others' needs, opinions, and attitudes. Criticism can send him in search of a candy bar, potato chips, and soda. Common emotional triggers for eating in the absence of physiological hunger are anxiety, depression, boredom, loneliness, fear, stress, excitement, joy, happiness, and many others. Food is the emotional eater's drug of choice, and instead of turning to less acceptable methods (such as drinking, gambling, or smoking) of dealing with life's curveballs, he heads for the freezer. All people, dieters at the top of the list, can fall quickly into emotional eating patterns, especially if they are overworked, deprived of quality sleep, or faced with more than they feel capable of handling.

Natural Eating *"Food is Not an issue"*

Natural eaters are the embodiment of the age-old nutrition tenets of variety, balance, and moderation. Natural eaters come in all shapes and sizes. Some are tall, lean, and lanky; others are round and soft; still others are muscular and solidly built. The common thread among natural eaters is that food is simply not an issue. They rarely think about food apart from designated meal and snack times and are able to eat a wide variety of foods—including so-called "junk foods"—without experiencing a moral dilemma. This often prompts their dieting acquaintances to remark "How can you finish that *whole* slice of cheesecake?! I'd feel so guilty!" or "How can you eat whatever you want and never gain an ounce?" or "What do you mean, 'you don't want a brownie right now'?"

Do you know people who seem to be natural eaters? Spend time with them, observe their behavior, and listen to their conversations. You won't hear them talking about the latest, greatest fad diet or discussing the calorie, fat, or carbohydrate content of the foods being served as if that were the most fascinating topic of the day. Natural eaters have a knack for listening to their bodies, honoring what they know about nutrition, and respecting their own and others' food preferences. Sound appealing? There's a natural eater inside each and every person waiting to be discovered. Resolve here and now never to tread the dieting path again; life has so much more to offer!

Respond to Hunger and Respect Natural Boundaries: Taming the Beast

One of the most concrete steps you can take to uncover your natural eater is also one of the most basic—respond to your unique body's signals that ask for nourishment. People who have ignored these signals for much of their adult lives often report that their appetites resemble insatiable beasts instead of the gifts that they truly are. This can be a direct result of past dieting or attempts at severe calorie restriction. In a classic study on the implications of starvation, Ancel Keys and his colleagues made intriguing observations of men who voluntarily restricted calorie intake to half their typical levels (*Biology of Human Starvation*, University of Minnesota Press, 1950). Among other disturbing characteristics, the subjects enrolled in the study displayed

- Food obsession—These men spent most of their waking hours contemplating food, recipes, eating, meals, snacks, and calories. They talked about food, collected recipes, and fantasized about elaborate meals that included their favorite foods.
- Compulsive eating behavior—They hoarded food, pushed food around on their plates to prolong meals, and binged when they were allowed free access to food during the "re-feeding" period of the study.
- Depressed cognitive function—Subjects were apathetic, despondent, tired, and uninterested in sexual activity. They could no longer think creatively.

Does any of this sound eerily familiar? Normal, everyday people can exhibit the same characteristics when they consciously restrict calories to a level that is inadequate for daily activities and functions. Learn to work *with*, not against, your body's physiological hunger signals to optimize your health and quality of life. Many people find it useful, at least in the beginning, to think of their level of hunger or fullness on a scale similar to the one in Figure 3.2.

FIGURE 3.2

The Hunger-Fullness Scale helps you clarify internal signals.

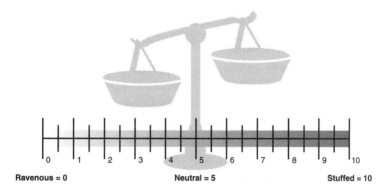

Ravenous = 0   Neutral = 5   Stuffed = 10

0—absolutely famished

1—extremely hungry

2—very hungry

3—hungry

4—just beginning to feel hungry

5—neither hungry nor satisfied

6—just beginning to feel satisfied

7—comfortably satisfied

8—full

9—extremely full

10—stuffed or nauseous

If this is the first time you've made an effort to identify your body's hunger signals, don't worry about doing it "correctly." Each person experiences hunger and fullness a little differently, and there are no rules about how often and how much you should eat. Some people prefer to allow themselves to get fairly hungry in between meal times; they tend toward the traditional "three squares" a day. Others don't like getting that hungry and would rather eat smaller amounts more frequently; they are often called *grazers*. Both styles of eaters are legitimately honoring their bodies' signals. It will be up to you to determine the best way to incorporate responding to your hunger in your particular lifestyle.

Chapters 4, "Balanced Nutrition," and 5, "Putting It Together—Real Food for Real People," address what to eat to honor your taste buds and your overall health. For now, just concentrate on making eating a priority when you become hungry.

If you're thinking "What kind of plan is this? Eat when I'm hungry?! What if I can't stop? I need concrete rules!" take a deep breath (or 10 or 20) and relax. It's taken a long time to get where you are today, and it may take a long time to become comfortable with the natural eating process. Expect it to be a learning experience, complete with mistakes, blunders, and a healthy dose of humility. As you're learning to respond to your body's hunger signals, you'll also want to start tuning in to your body's satiety, or fullness, signals, which are also illustrated in Figure 3.2. Varying levels of satiety correspond with numbers 6 through 10 on the Hunger-Fullness Scale. To respond to these signals, you will need to become more mindful during the eating process.

Mindfulness: The Art of Eating

Mindfulness, or paying attention, is a technique inherent in the natural eater. It sounds so simple, doesn't it? But in a world that pushes convenience, speed, and efficiency, paying attention to what, how much, when, and why you eat can be daunting. The following concepts can help you work toward a more mindful eating experience.

Know That You Can Eat Again

If you believe that this is the last time you will enjoy steak and potatoes (at least for a while), you create a mindset that lends itself to overeating. As you recall from the study on human starvation, deprivation usually promotes binging when food becomes available again. Overeating is not a sign of a defect in character; rather, it often points to prior restriction of food or particular types of food. This is why diets that place certain foods on "to be avoided" lists almost never work in the long haul.

Make Eating a Priority

It's difficult to be mindful when you're trying to eat, talk on a cell phone, and navigate the morning rush hour. Even if you have only five minutes to devote to a meal, sit down, take a deep breath, and enjoy it as much as possible. If your food options are limited, make the best of the situation and focus on whatever is sitting in front of you.

Create a Positive Eating Atmosphere

Many people find it helpful to go out of their way to create a positive, relaxed atmosphere when they eat. You've probably heard it before, but this time act on it! Go ahead—get out the candles, put on good music, use real flatware, turn off the TV, and don't answer the phone (or email or voice mail). This particular concept takes many different forms depending on your needs and preferences. Some people find cleanup after meals to be such a burden that they occasionally use disposable plates and utensils to feel more relaxed while they're eating. These aren't rules, merely suggestions. Do whatever you can do to eat in a positive environment.

Honor Your Taste Buds

Have you ever eaten a food strictly for its health-promoting qualities? I've worked with many clients who consistently order a salad for lunch, dutifully munch through a plate that sometimes contains far more calories than they realize, and get absolutely no satisfaction from that meal. What happens in the afternoons? They raid the vending machine or a colleague's candy dish for food that tastes good to them. By respecting your unique food preferences and choosing to eat a variety of foods that you truly enjoy at mealtime, you will be less likely to go on food raids at other times of the day.

Check In with Your Body During the Meal

This is especially helpful if you have little control over the portions served, as in restaurant meals. As soon as you are served, mentally or physically separate the meal into two or more portions. When you've finished one portion, pause for a moment to evaluate how you feel, how the food tastes, and if you really want the rest. If you're eating at home, you can accomplish this "body check-in" by starting with smaller servings, eating what's on your plate, pausing for a short break, and then deciding whether to get another helping. Sometimes you may choose to keep eating, even if you know that you have had enough to satisfy your physiological hunger. Special meals or celebrations and traveling to places that offer new foods are common and legitimate reasons to eat more than usual. The key is to recognize that your body and appetite will adjust for these decisions, and your next hunger signals may not appear as soon as they usually do!

As you become a more mindful eater, it may become clear that you are or have been using food to meet legitimate, nonhunger needs.

Understand and Meet Your *Other* Needs

Hunger is one of the most primal drives that humans experience, but it certainly isn't the only need to which you must attend. Far too many people attempt to use food to meet these other needs, often to the detriment of their overall health and well-being. Part of leading a balanced lifestyle includes being able to identify and satisfy some basic needs in an appropriate manner. These needs include, but are not limited to

- Adequate, quality sleep
- Physical activity
- Appropriate medical care
- Connecting with other people (emotionally, physically, spiritually, intellectually, and socially)

■ Expressing emotions and thoughts

■ Respect

■ Rewards

■ Pleasure

■ Relaxation

How about you? Do you look to food to manage these needs? Do you eat when you are tired? Stressed? Bored? Lonely? Anxious? Do you reward yourself with food? Do you feel like you haven't taken a legitimate break from work unless you've had something to eat? Is food your primary sensual pleasure?

If you've answered yes to some or most of these questions, it's time to take a serious look at your behaviors and evaluate how you can begin meeting these needs in a healthier way. It never hurts to talk to someone you trust or to seek out a qualified counselor to help you identify and develop ways of satisfying your legitimate needs as a human being. The following story shows how one of my clients learned how to meet her own needs and break an emotional eating pattern.

Managing Emotional Eating (Gail's Story)

One of nine children growing up on a farm, Gail recalls childhood meals full of fried foods and unlimited desserts. Though body weight was "part of my family's consciousness," neither Gail nor any of her family members were seriously overweight, due in part to working the farm and plenty of bicycling on country roads. Throughout her high school years, however, Gail began to struggle more and more with her body image, self-confidence, and eating patterns.

"I don't remember having very much fun in high school. A couple of my older sisters had gotten into trouble, so I tried to be the perfect student. I got a job, dated a little, and went to night school, and that was the first time I can remember dieting. I know now that I was bulimic, but we didn't call it that at the time. I remember stopping eating for six days at one point; I was thin, but I was totally out of control."

Fortunately, Gail recognized how unhealthy she had become and gradually stopped her purging behaviors, going on to marry and move to Indianapolis. The move proved stressful, and she again turned to eating to manage her emotions. At 36, Gail was diagnosed with osteoarthritis and placed on medications, while her work environment and one particular supervisor were driving her back to destructive eating patterns.

"It was a horrible situation, and I started eating to deal with my unhappiness. I probably gained 50 pounds that year."

After discontinuing her arthritis medications during pregnancy, Gail decided she didn't want to start them up again after she'd delivered her son, so she joined the NIFS Fitness Center in 1996.

"I knew it needed to be convenient and supportive, and it was, but I was really disappointed that I didn't lose weight quickly at first. I yo-yo'd up and down for about seven years before I finally decided I had had enough. On December 4, 2002, I had just gotten to the point where I was feeling really horrible. I had watched a TV program that encouraged people to seek out a support system and develop goals, so that night, I drew up my own personal timeline. My goal was to lose 40 pounds, one pound per week."

Gail still struggled with emotional eating and with finding a time for her workouts, but she had an "a-ha" moment with both issues. First, she decided to keep track of every situation or emotion that seemed to trigger negative eating patterns. She wrote each situation on an index card, and on the reverse side, developed a list of "eating alternatives" for that particular situation.

I carried those cards with me wherever I went—in the car, at work, in my purse. They were always there to remind me what to do if I was struggling."

As for finding time for her workouts, Gail decided to juggle her schedule a bit to move exercise to her lunch "hour."

"It just came to me. I asked my boss if I could come in a little earlier and stay a little later, and take a long lunch for my midday workouts. I'm still coming to NIFS almost every day during the week to exercise. I know how important it is for stress relief, and it's almost like I have two days within a day now. I get to shower and go back to work in the afternoon more refreshed."

Gail firmly believes in personal responsibility for changing your habits while finding support and accountability to help you accomplish your goals.

"You have to find that place or that group or that person to support you—something to provide the consistency and accountability. It's tough to get out of the destructive cycles; I know I couldn't have done it without my husband.

But you have to make the decision. No one else can do it for you. I know my body so much better now. I know how I feel when I eat too much, and, because I'm much more tuned in to my body, I just don't think I'll ever go back to the kind of patterns I had before."

Natural Eating Starts Now

This is a perfect time in the process to evaluate your overall relationship with food. Is it generally positive? Do you tend to eat in response to internal cues rather than environmental, social, and emotional cues? If you feel like you have a long way to go, focus on making the transition to natural eating before you continue with the remaining chapters in this book. Even the most sound nutrition advice can become "diet-like" when applied inappropriately. Focus on healing your relationship with food before you tackle more specific nutrition information—you'll be healthier, happier, and more confident because of it!

THE ABSOLUTE MINIMUM

- The goal of natural eating is to create harmony between your needs for energy, pleasure, satisfaction, flexibility, and nourishment.

- Examine how you use food before you try to change what you eat.

- Responding to your body's hunger and fullness signals is the most basic form of natural eating.

- Get professional help if you think you're using food to fulfill other needs, and you can't determine how to identify those needs or meet them appropriately.

In This Chapter

- Balance the calories you consume with the calories you burn
- Understand the importance of fueling your body with carbohydrate, protein, and fat
- Understand the importance of fiber and get the lowdown on cholesterol
- Learn what vitamins and minerals can and cannot do

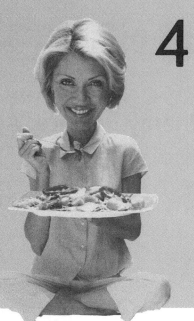

4

Balanced Nutrition

A healthy lifestyle and good nutrition are truly about *balance*—balance food and activity; balance nutritious and not-so-nutritious food choices; and balance the nutrients in your meals and snacks. In Chapter 3, "Uncover the Natural Eater," you learned about respecting your body's signals of hunger and fullness. In this chapter, you'll learn about each of the nutrients your body requires and will be better able to sift through the nutrition advice you get from a variety of avenues—some credible, others not so.

As you read, keep in mind some concepts to preserve your sanity and your trust in nutrition professionals as a whole. First, understand that nutrition is an evolving science, so don't be alarmed, upset, or surprised when nutrition recommendations change slightly or are updated by reputable organizations and individuals. Second, try not to assign value to foods. Some are more nutritious than others, but that doesn't make them "good" or "bad." Finally, know that *you* are the ultimate decision maker when it comes to what passes your lips—not me, not another dietitian, and certainly not an impersonal (albeit reputable) organization. This chapter is about information—you decide how much or little you're ready to implement in your own life!

Energy Balance: An Enigmatic Equation

Although you cannot change your genetic makeup, you do have some manner of control over energy intake and expenditure. Many people get hung up on trying to achieve the perfect combination of carbohydrate, fat, and protein and neglect the basic tenet of calorie balance. In a comprehensive review of literature, however, researchers concluded that energy restriction (lowering calorie intake) was the only variable that correlated with weight loss (*J Am Diet Assoc. 2001; 101:411–420*).

note

In theory, one pound of body fat contains approximately 3,500 calories of stored energy. Therefore, a 500-calorie deficit per day (500 calories × 7 days per week = 3,500 calories) will yield one pound of fat loss per week.

It seems so straightforward on paper, doesn't it? In reality, things may not be so simple. In other studies in which subjects voluntarily consume far more calories than they would under normal conditions, they do gain weight but not nearly as much as the numbers indicate. In other words, their bodies adjust to the higher calorie intake and begin burning calories like it's going out of style! In much the same way, when people restrict calories to a level dramatically lower than usual (as they commonly do when trying to lose weight), their bodies adjust by burning calories more slowly. Do they lose weight? Yes, but probably not as much as a straight numbers analysis would predict. The bottom line is that your body will go to great lengths to remain at a stable weight, regardless of your actual calorie intake. So what's the take-home message? If you want to change your weight and your life for good, focus on the habits, attitudes, and situations that *influence* the calories you consume and burn instead of on the calories themselves. It certainly doesn't hurt to be aware of the calorie content of the foods you commonly eat, especially those you consume outside the home, but don't get caught in a numbers game.

There are ways of measuring energy expenditure directly, but most are costly and time consuming. You can get a rough estimate of your daily calorie needs by walking through the following steps instead. The total calories you burn each day can be broken into three main compartments—*basal* calorie needs, calories for *physical activity*, and calories for the *thermic effect of food*. Basal calories cover your energy needs at rest and keep vital organs such as your brain, heart, lungs, kidneys, and liver functioning. The majority (about 60%) of your total daily calorie needs fulfill your basal energy requirements. You can estimate your basal calorie needs by multiplying your healthy body weight in pounds by 10:

> Healthy body weight (lbs.) × 10 = Basal calorie needs

Example:

Sandra currently weighs 175 lbs. and has determined that her comfortable, healthy weight is around 160 lbs. She walks for 30 minutes two to three times a week and has a sedentary job:

> *160 lbs × 10 = 1,600 calories for basal needs*

Most people also need calories for daily activity—if not for exercise, then for showering, getting dressed, taking care of children, or going to work. If you are sedentary or only minimally active, the calories you need for physical activity compose about 30% or less of your total daily needs. Very active individuals may spend up to 50% or more of their total daily calories on physical activity! Add calories for physical activity to your total daily needs by multiplying your basal calories by one of the following factors:

- 1.2 if you are sedentary
- 1.3 if you are lightly active (easy walking, swimming, or biking a few times a week; or your job involves light activity)
- 1.4 if you are moderately active (planned exercise most days of the week at a fairly challenging intensity)
- 1.5 or more if you are very active (intense exercise most days of the week or a physically demanding job—for example, construction worker)

> Basal calorie needs × activity factor = basal calories + calories for physical activity

Example, continued:

> *1,600 calories × 1.3 = 2,080 calories for basal needs and physical activity*

The final compartment of energy expenditure is the thermic effect of food. These are the calories your body uses to process the food you eat. This forms only a small percentage (10 or less) of your total daily calorie needs. Add thermic effect of food calories to the total by multiplying your answer from earlier by 1.1:

> (Basal calories + calories for physical activity) × 1.1 = Total Daily Calorie Needs

Example, continued:

> *2,080 calories × 1.1 = 2,288 calories per day for weight maintenance*

If Sandra wanted to lose weight gradually and healthfully, she could increase her physical activity and reduce her calorie intake to around 2,000 calories per day.

Are you tired of math? Don't sweat it. As you learned early in this section, it is counterproductive to focus exclusively on calories while improving your lifestyle. Your body does an amazing job of balancing the energy it burns with the amount you consume through food. Focus instead on improving the nutritional *value* of the calories you consume, and that will leave plenty of room for enjoying some foods purely for pleasure!

Macronutrients: Fuel for Working Bodies

Three nutrients are responsible for providing your body with energy, or calories—carbohydrate, protein, and fat. Because you need relatively large amounts of these nutrients, they are called *macronutrients*. Each of the macronutrients has specific functions in your body, but in some cases, one can be interchanged with another. A perfect example of this takes place during exercise. Working muscles prefer to use carbohydrates for energy, but in a pinch (if you haven't eaten enough carbohydrate-rich foods or if you've exhausted the supply in your muscles), fat can provide energy as well. Read on to discover how your body depends on each of these important nutrients!

Carbohydrates: Energy for Muscles and Minds

Carbohydrates are composed of units of carbon, hydrogen, and oxygen (commonly referred to as units of *sugar*) and are the body's principle source of energy, providing about four calories per gram. Most carbohydrates are eventually converted to glucose or glycogen in your body. Your central nervous system, including your brain, relies almost exclusively on glucose for fuel, and your muscles are powered primarily by glycogen during activity—two compelling reasons to make carbohydrate-rich foods a staple of your diet! In fact, 45% to 65% of your total calories should come from carbohydrates (in general, the more active you are, the more carbohydrate calories you require). This macronutrient comes in two forms—simple and complex.

Simple carbohydrates are those that consist of just one or two units of sugar. They are found naturally in fruit, fruit juices, and milk—all of which contain other important nutrients—and are added to many foods in processing. Table sugar, honey, syrups, candy, cookies, ice cream, fruit-flavored beverages, and colas are all examples of foods high in simple carbohydrates that provide calories but few additional nutrients.

Complex carbohydrates consist of many units of sugar and are often referred to as *starches*. Grain and plant foods such as cereals, pastas, rice, bread, crackers, potatoes, corn, and beans are all rich in complex carbohydrates as well as vitamins, minerals, water, and dietary fiber. Most of these foods are also naturally low in fat.

You can estimate your daily need for grams of carbohydrates by multiplying your total daily calorie needs by your desired percentage of calories from carbohydrates (45% to 65%—less if you're sedentary; more if you're active) and dividing that number by four (there are four calories per gram of carbohydrate):

Total daily calories × ____% = Calories from carbohydrate

Calories from carbohydrate ÷ 4 calories per gram = Grams of carbohydrate needed per day

Example (continuing with Sandra from earlier example):

2,000 calories per day × 0.50 (50%) = 1,000 calories from carbohydrate

1,000 calories ÷ 4 calories per gram = 250 grams of carbohydrate per day

---

WHY NOT GO LOW CARB?

The popularity of low carbohydrate diets is causing quite a stir among health professionals, government organizations, and ordinary people trying to figure out the best way to lose weight. Unfortunately, these diets ignore some of the most fundamental issues regarding unhealthy body weight: an abundance of high-calorie, nutrient-sparse foods; lack of physical activity; unmanaged stress; and inadequate coping skills. *Any* diet that manipulates food choices to reduce total calorie intake has a good chance of producing weight loss, and cutting back on carbohydrate-rich foods is a pretty simple way of accomplishing just that. Most studies, however, show that the *composition* of those calories is not as important as the sheer *number* in determining weight loss. The bottom line is that diets of any kind promote distorted relationships with food, eating, and your body. You are taught that you can't trust yourself with certain types of foods, that these foods are prohibited, and that if you "cheat," you must pay a heavy price…hardly the kind of thought process conducive to overall mental, emotional, and physical health. Do yourself a favor and learn how to eat all foods, including those high in carbohydrates, in moderate amounts.

Fabulous Fiber

Fiber is an indigestible carbohydrate found only in plant foods that deserves special mention because of its health-promoting properties. Fruits, vegetables, whole-grain products, beans, peas, nuts, and seeds are all good sources of fiber. Adults need anywhere from 21 to 38 grams of fiber daily, depending on gender and calorie needs. See Table 4.1 to determine your daily fiber recommendations.

TABLE 4.1 Your Daily Fiber Needs

Gender	Age	Grams of Fiber
Male	under 50	38 grams
	over 50	30 grams
Female	under 50	25 grams
	over 50	21 grams

There are two types of fiber—soluble and insoluble. Each type confers different health benefits. *Soluble fiber* forms a gel in water and is responsible for improving blood cholesterol levels. It may also be useful in controlling blood sugar levels— particularly important for people with diabetes. *Insoluble fiber* does not form a gel in water and can help keep your digestive system working properly and may help prevent colon cancer. Fiber-rich foods contain a combination of both types of fiber, but one often occurs in a higher proportion. See Table 4.2 for some of the most common food sources of each type of fiber.

TABLE 4.2 Common Food Sources of Soluble and Insoluble Fiber

Type of Fiber	Food Sources
Soluble	Oats and related products (oatmeal, oat bran, or foods made from them), barley, cooked legumes (dried beans, peas, and lentils), many fruits, and some vegetables
Insoluble	Whole grains and their products, wheat bran, many vegetables, some fruits, nuts, seeds, and brown rice

WHY WHOLE GRAINS?

Whole grains and their related food products are nutrition powerhouses. Unfortunately, many of the grain foods we eat have been processed in a way that removes vital nutrients. What's the difference, and how can you tell whether you're buying a whole grain? The original grain has three main components—the bran, endosperm, and germ (see Figure 4.1). Food processors often remove the bran and the germ, so that the resulting product may be deficient in the nutrients concentrated in those parts of the grain. Refined grains tend to be lower in fiber, B vitamins, and some minerals than their whole-grain counterparts. To determine whether you are purchasing a whole-grain bread, cereal, bagel, pasta, or other product, look at the ingredient list for the word "whole"—it should appear *early* in the list (preferably first). Words such as "cracked," "enriched," "nine grain," "wheat," and others often appear on bread and cracker labels, but don't necessarily indicate a true whole grain.

FIGURE 4.1
Anatomy of a
whole grain.

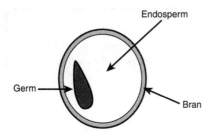

Protein Power

Protein provides about four calories per gram, similar to carbohydrate, and is an essential component of virtually thousands of substances in your body. Cells, tissues, hormones, and enzymes all rely on protein for their building blocks. Protein also plays a key role in fluid balance and immune function. The newest recommendations from the National Academy of Sciences suggest that protein can provide from 10% to 35% of your total calorie intake. This relatively wide range illustrates differences in individual protein needs. You can estimate your own needs in one of several ways:

- Method 1—As a percentage of your total calorie needs
- Method 2—Based on healthy body weight in kilograms (per Recommended Dietary Allowance)
- Method 3—Based on body weight in pounds and activity level

For simplicity's sake, use Method 3 in Figure 4.2 to get a rough estimate of your protein needs.

Protein is present in many foods. Lean meats, poultry, fish, eggs, and dairy products are common animal sources of protein. However, beans, lentils, peas, soy products, nuts, and seeds also provide protein, are low in cholesterol and saturated fats, and are rich in other important nutrients.

note

A registered dietitian (RD) can help you determine your protein needs more accurately based on your health history, goals, and personal preferences.

FIGURE 4.2

Estimating your daily protein needs.

Sedentary (little daily activity through exercise or occupation)
→ 0.4 to 0.5 grams per pound of body weight

Moderately Active (exercise 3 to 5 days per week at a moderate intensity) → 0.5 to 0.7 grams per pound of body weight

Very Active (exercise 6 to 7 days per week at a challenging intensity OR physically demanding occupation) → 0.7 to 1.0 grams per pound of body weight

EXAMPLE:

(Continuing with Sandra from earlier):
Sandra is probably on the low end of moderately active, so
multiply her body weight in pounds by 0.5 to 0.6 grams protein
to estimate her daily needs.
175 lbs X 0.5 to 0.6 grams protein = 88 to 105 grams protein
per day

The Skinny on Fat

Fat, once eschewed by health-conscious people everywhere, is coming back into fashion. It's important to recognize, however, that just like carbohydrate and protein, fat has always been essential for good health. Each gram of fat provides about 9 calories, so it's easy to see how foods rich in fat can bump up your total calorie intake quickly. Fat improves the taste of many foods; helps prolong feelings of satiety; and is critical for proper nerve conduction, production of hormones and cell walls, and absorption of fat-soluble vitamins (A, D, E, and K). Balance is important! Some fat, but not too much, is the key. Fat should provide about 20% to 35% of your total calorie intake. This range reflects differences in cultural and personal preferences, health needs, and levels of physical activity among individuals.

You can estimate your daily need for fat in grams in the same way you determined your carbohydrate needs. Start by multiplying your total daily calories by your desired percentage of calories from fat (20% to 35%). Then divide that number by 9 (because fat has 9 calories per gram) to obtain the number of grams of fat you'll consume each day:

> Total daily calories × ____% = Calories from fat
>
> Calories from fat ÷ 9 = Daily grams of fat

Example, continued:

> *2,000 calories per day × .30 (30%) = 600 calories from fat*
>
> *600 calories ÷ 9 calories per gram = 67 grams of fat per day*

Alternatively, you can calculate your carbohydrate and protein needs first, and then determine how many grams of fat are required to make up the balance of your daily calorie needs.

Many people consume more fat than necessary by relying too heavily on convenience foods and restaurants. Although keeping tabs on your total fat intake makes good sense, it's also important to realize that not all fats are created equally. Some types are associated with heart disease, cancer, diabetes, and other chronic illnesses, whereas others have been shown to *reduce* your risk for these very conditions. By understanding the health effects and food sources of different types of fats (see Figure 4.3), you can make informed decisions about your meals and snacks.

TRANS FATS: FRIEND OR FOE?

Trans fatty acids are formed when unsaturated liquid vegetable oils are hydrogenated (hydrogen atoms are added) to create a product with a longer shelf life. Although trans fatty acids occur naturally in some animal fats, the majority of the trans fat we consume comes from packaged foods such as crackers, chips, and baked goods: fried foods; stick margarine; and shortening.

Current research shows that trans fatty acids can increase your risk for heart disease by raising LDL (bad) cholesterol and lowering HDL (good) cholesterol (see the section

"Concerned About Cholesterol?" following this sidebar for an explanation of these terms). How can you decrease your intake of trans fatty acids? Try the following:

- Minimize your consumption of processed foods containing *hydrogenated* or *partially hydrogenated* anything. Read the ingredient list on food labels; some products also list trans fats on the nutrition facts panel. By 2006, manufacturers will be required to list trans fats in grams on all products.

- Go easy on the French fries and any other fried dishes when dining out. Some restaurants and fast food places fry foods in hydrogenated vegetable oils that contain trans fatty acids.

- If you use margarine, choose a spray, squeeze, or soft tub variety over stick margarine. Many of these products are labeled *trans fat free.*

- Prepare more meals and snacks at home with whole, fresh foods!

FIGURE 4.3

Understanding four main types of fats.

Type	Function	Food Sources	Health Effects	Tips
Mono-unsaturated	Structural component of cell membranes, especially the coating of nerve cells	Most plant sources; olive oil, canola oil, and peanut oil; nuts, seeds, avocados, and olives	May decrease LDL-(bad) cholesterol; no effect on HDL-(good) cholesterol	Substitute these fats for saturated fats whenever possible.
Poly-unsaturated	Precursor for hormones; component of cell membranes; essential for normal growth and development	Omega-3: salmon, mackerel, tuna, walnuts, flaxseed and flaxseed oil, canola oil	May lower LDL-, no effect on HDL- cholesterol	These fats may also help reduce inflammation and blood clotting.
		Omega-6: safflower, corn, sunflower and soybean oils, mayonnaise, commercial salad dressing	May lower both LDL- and HDL- cholesterol	Most of us get plenty of omega-6 fatty acids; focus on omega-3s instead.
Saturated	Structural component of cell membranes; provides desirable taste and texture in foods	Most animal foods, whole and reduced fat milk products, many desserts, baked goods, snack foods, coconut oil, palm oil and palm kernel oil	May increase LDL- and HDL- cholesterol	Limit this fat by choosing skim milk products, lean meats, and more plant-based proteins.
Trans	No essential functions	Any food containing the ingredients "hydrogenated or partially hydrogenated" oils, most processed or packaged foods, stick margarine, fast foods	May increase LDL- and decrease HDL- cholesterol	Try to reduce intake of trans fats as much as possible; prepare more meals and snacks at home.

Concerned About Cholesterol?

Cholesterol is a white, waxy, fatlike substance that is an important component of hormones and cell walls in your body. Your liver produces all the cholesterol you need, so it really isn't a dietary necessity. Many people have the ability to regulate cholesterol production in the liver based on the amount they obtain from food each day. If you're one of the lucky ones, you may eat foods rich in cholesterol, but your blood levels stay relatively constant because the liver simply produces less cholesterol. In others, however, this mechanism doesn't work quite as well, and the liver just keeps churning out cholesterol regardless of the amount obtained from food.

Because there is no simple way to determine into which of these two categories you fall, health professionals usually recommend that healthy people try to limit their cholesterol intake to 300mg per day or less; those who are at high risk for cardiovascular disease or who already have elevated blood cholesterol should limit their dietary intake to 200mg per day or less. Cholesterol is found only in animal products and is highest in foods such as egg yolks, organ meats such as liver or brain, red meats, poultry skin, some shellfish, and regular dairy products (cheese, ice cream, cream, butter, and so on).

A *blood lipid panel* can provide information about the levels of total cholesterol, *HDL (high-density lipoprotein) cholesterol*, *LDL (low-density lipoprotein) cholesterol*, and *triglycerides*. HDL, or "helpful" cholesterol, removes cholesterol from the blood and body tissues and transports it to the liver to be processed, whereas LDL, or "lousy" cholesterol, takes cholesterol from the liver and bloodstream and deposits it in blood vessels and body tissues. High LDL and total cholesterol and low HDL levels are associated with an increased risk for cardiovascular disease. Triglycerides are the most dominant form of fatty acids in the body, and elevated blood levels of these fats may indicate an increased risk for cardiovascular disease as well. See Appendix A, "Worksheets and Additional Resources," for information about desirable levels for all these health indices.

Micronutrients Keep the Machine Running Smoothly

Think of vitamins and minerals, or *micronutrients*, as the body's "spark plugs" and "motor oil." They are responsible for jump starting the reactions that take place at the level of individual cells in your body and for making sure that these reactions run smoothly. They do not, contrary to popular belief, provide energy; rather, they help your body utilize the energy that it gets from macronutrients. It's best to obtain vitamins and minerals from the foods you eat for several reasons. First, foods contain exquisite combinations of nutrients that may enhance the absorption of those nutrients in ways we don't yet fully understand. Second, foods contain thousands of substances, many of which have yet to be discovered, that may positively influence your health. Third, the supplement industry is poorly regulated, so it's difficult to determine the quality, safety, and efficacy of the product. Besides, eating food is just more fun than popping pills!

THINKING ABOUT SUPPLEMENTS?

If so, the phrase of the day is "buyer beware." The supplement industry is essentially unregulated, which means that manufacturers do not have to show proof of their product's safety or efficacy to take it to market. There are some ethical, reputable manufacturers, and, unfortunately, many that are not so. Your best bet is to stick with a standard multivitamin and mineral supplement that contains no more than 100% of the daily value for any recognized nutrient—information that should appear on every package on the supplement facts panel. Contrary to popular belief, getting more than 100% of your daily needs for vitamins and minerals through supplements does not provide greater benefit, and in some cases, can cause unpleasant or serious side effects. Specific populations may benefit from individual supplements, but talk to your physician and/or a registered dietitian before you spend your hard-earned money on any of them.

Vitamins

Vitamins are organic substances that help regulate cell functions; they are classified as either fat-soluble (A, D, E, and K) or water-soluble (the B vitamins and vitamin C). *Fat-soluble vitamins* can be stored in the body's fat tissue for relatively long periods of time, whereas *water-soluble vitamins* are usually flushed out through the urine and need to be replenished frequently.

Minerals

Minerals are elements used in the body to regulate chemical reactions and form body structures. They are found in a wide variety of foods and are classified as major or trace minerals based on the amount you need daily. The major minerals include sodium, potassium, chloride, calcium, phosphorus, magnesium, and sulfur. The trace minerals include iron, zinc, copper, selenium, iodide, fluoride, chromium, manganese, and molybdenum. Eating a variety of foods maximizes your chances of consuming adequate amounts of minerals.

SODIUM, SALT, AND SUCH

Sodium is a mineral needed by your body in small amounts (probably only about 500mg daily) for electrolyte and fluid balance and for transmitting nerve impulses. The newest recommendation from the National Academy of Sciences is to limit your sodium intake to 1,500mg per day or less, but most people easily consume many times this amount. Some individuals are sodium sensitive, meaning high sodium intake contributes to high blood pressure, and low sodium intake may correct high blood pressure. It's interesting to note, however, that some cultures with very high intakes of sodium also have low incidences of hypertension and heart disease, so the puzzle is far from complete.

Sodium is found naturally in some foods, but most of your intake comes from processed food or eating in restaurants where you don't have much control over food preparation. Another common source of sodium is the salt shaker—just one teaspoon of the white stuff contains about 2,000 milligrams of sodium. Some common names of ingredients high in sodium include sodium chloride, monosodium glutamate (MSG), brine, baking soda, broth, bouillon, and soy sauce. Read food labels to identify hidden sources of sodium and try some or all of the following to reduce your sodium intake if you, your physician, or a registered dietitian determines this to be a prudent step. Keep in mind that the taste for sodium is learned and takes some time to unlearn. Make changes gradually to avoid the "this tastes like cardboard" syndrome!

- Cook foods without adding salt. Experiment with spices and herbs to give dishes more flavor. Add salt just before serving if needed.
- Limit high sodium condiments such as soy sauce, marinades, ketchup, and mustard. Try fresh tomatoes, lettuce, and chopped onion instead.
- Purchase No Added Salt canned or frozen vegetables, or focus on using the fresh veggies in your crisper drawer.
- Rinse canned vegetables and beans under water in a colander to remove much of the sodium.
- Limit cured, pickled, and processed foods such as bacon, ham, pickles, luncheon meats, salty chips and snacks, and frozen meals and snacks.
- If you do purchase packaged foods, look for those labeled *sodium free*, *low* or *very low in sodium*, *reduced sodium*, *unsalted*, or *no added salt*.
- Prepare more foods at home to decrease reliance on packaged foods!

Micronutrients are a complex and often confusing subject. Figures 4.4 and 4.5 provide more detailed information on specific functions and food sources of key vitamins and minerals.

FIGURE 4.4

Understanding vitamins.

NAME	RDA/AI*	FUNCTION	SOURCE
Vitamin A	700 ug (F) 900 ug (M)	Vision, growth, prevent drying of skin and eyes, promote resistance to infection	Liver, fortified milk, yams, spinach, carrots, apricots, cantaloupe, broccoli
Riboflavin	1.1 mg (F) 1.3 mg (M)	Essential for growth, energy metabolism	Milk, mushrooms, spinach, liver, enriched grains
Thiamin	1.1 mg (F) 1.2 mg (M)	Metabolism, nerve function	Sunflower seeds, lean meats, whole and enriched grains, peas
Niacin	14 mg (F) 16 mg (M)	Energy metabolism, fat synthesis and breakdown	Bran, fish, beef, chicken, peanuts, enriched grains
Folate	400 ug	DNA and RNA synthesis, amino acid synthesis, decrease risk of birth defects	Leafy greens, citrus fruits, whole and enriched grains, beans, orange juice, fortified cereals
Vitamin B6	1.3 mg 19-50yrs 1.5 mg (F > 50 yrs) 1.7 mg (M > 50 yrs)	Protein metabolism, hemoglobin synthesis	Animal protein foods, broccoli, bananas, beans, whole grains, citrus fruits
Vitamin B12	2.4 ug	Nerve function, red blood cell metabolism	Dairy products, chicken, pork, shellfish, beef
Vitamin C	75 mg (F) 90 mg (M) Add 35 mg for smokers	Collagen, hormone, and neurotransmitter synthesis, wound healing, iron absorption	Citrus fruits, strawberries, broccoli, greens, potatoes
Vitamin D	200 IU 19-50 yrs 400 IU 50-70 yrs 600 IU > 70 yrs	Facilitate absorption of calcium and phosphorous, maintain bone calcium	Fortfied milk, sardines, salmon, produced by body in response to sunlight
Vitamin E	15 mg	Antioxidant: prevent break-down of vitamin A and unsaturated fatty acids	Vegetable oils, wheat germ, peanuts, leafy greens, seeds
Vitamin K	90 ug (F) 120 ug (M)	Blood clotting	Leafy greens, broccoli, eggs, soybeans

(F) = Females   (M) = Males   IU = International Units   mg = Milligrams   ug = Micrograms   RDA - Recommended Dietary Allowances
*Amounts given for persons aged 19-70 unless otherwise noted.   AI - Adequate Intakes

FIGURE 4.5

Understanding minerals.

NAME	RDA/AI*	FUNCTION	SOURCE
Iron	18 mg (F) 19-50 yrs 8 mg (M) 8 mg (F) > 50yrs	Hemoglobin, immune function	Meats, leafy greens, seafood, dried fruits, beans, fortified cerals, nuts
Calcium	1000 mg 19-50 yrs 1200 mg > 50 yrs	Bone and teeth formation, nerve transmission, muscle contraction	Dairy products, leafy greens, some tofu, canned fish with bones, fortified orange juice
Zinc	8 mg (F) 11 mg (M)	Enzyme function, wound healing, growth, immunity	Seafoods, meats, greens, beans, whole grains, eggs, poultry
Magnesium	310-320 mg (F) 400-420 mg (M)	Bones, nerve and heart function	Whole grains, legumes, tea, broccoli, nuts, beans, bananas, soy beans
Chromium	25 ug (F) 19 - 50 yrs 20 ug (F) > 50 yrs 35 ug (M) 19 - 50 yrs 30 ug (M) > 50 yrs	Metabolism of carbohydrates and fats	Whole grains, meat, cheese, egg yolk, fortified cereal, mushrooms
Sodium	≤ 1500 mg 19 - 50 yrs ≤ 1300 mg 50 - 70 yrs ≤ 1200 mg > 70 yrs	Electolyte and water balance, nerve transmission	Table salt, processed foods
Potassium	4700 mg	Electrolyte balance, nerve transmission	Bananas, meat, beans, orange juice, yogurt, potatoes
Phosphorous	700 mg	Bone and teeth formation, energy production	Dairy products, meat, fish, beans, sodas, eggs
Copper	900 ug	Aids in protein metabolism	Beans, nuts, whole grains, shellfish, dried fruits, cocoa
Selenium	55 ug	Antioxidant functions	Meats, fish, eggs, milk, seafood, whole grains
Manganese	1.8 mg (F) 2.3 mg (M)	Enzyme action including carbohydrate metabolism	Nuts, oats, beans, tea, rice, whole grains
Chloride	≤ 2300 mg 19 - 50 yrs ≤ 2000 mg 50 - 70 yrs ≤ 1800 mg > 70 yrs	Maintain fluid and acid-base balance	Table salt, processed foods, fish

(F) = Females   (M) = Males   mg = Milligrams   ug = Micrograms   RDA - Recommended Dietary Allowances
*Amounts given for persons aged 19-70 unless otherwise noted.   AI - Adequate Intakes

Water: The Beverage of Champions

Although water is not really a nutrient, it is so essential for human life that you can survive only a few days without it. Approximately two-thirds of your body is composed of water, and all cell processes and organ functions depend on it. Water also acts as a lubricant, moves food through the intestinal tract, and helps regulate body temperature. The standard recommendation is to drink eight 8-ounce glasses of water daily. This isn't a magic number, but it will ensure adequate hydration for most healthy people. If you are very active, or you sweat a lot, you may need much more water than the "eight 8-ounces" rule of thumb. Your need for water is closely related to your calorie intake—the more calories you consume, the more water your body requires. Now would be a good time to repeat the self-test you performed in Chapter 2, "The Stages of Change—What to Expect"—check the frequency and color of your urine. You should be voiding every two to three hours, and it should be fairly pale in color.

Liquid foods such as juice, milk, and soup can also contribute to fluid intake. Caffeinated beverages such as coffee, tea, and some colas may have a slight diuretic effect, which means they can cause loss of body water through increased urination. This effect is more pronounced in people who don't drink caffeinated beverages regularly. If you enjoy a cup or two of coffee or tea most mornings, you can consider them part of your total daily fluid needs without much concern.

THE ABSOLUTE MINIMUM

Okay, you made it through Nutrition 101—great job! This material laid the groundwork for Chapter 5, "Putting It Together—Real Food for Real People," by helping you understand the nutrients you'll obtain from foods you eat. Key points to remember:

■ Your body weight is a function of the calories you consume versus the calories you burn—to an extent.

■ Your body has clever ways of maintaining a stable weight, so don't obsess over calories.

■ Carbohydrate, protein, and fat (macronutrients) all play important roles in your healthy eating plan.

■ Vitamins and minerals (micronutrients) do not provide energy, but they do help your body utilize the energy it gets from the macronutrients.

■ Water isn't a nutrient per se, but you can't function properly without it—aim for eight 8-ounce glasses daily.

- A food guide pyramid primer—learn how to make it work for you

- Understand how food groups and serving sizes can help you meet your nutrition needs

- Translate this information into quick, tasty, and nutritious meals

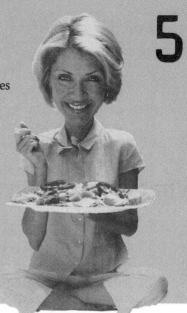

5

PUTTING IT TOGETHER— REAL FOOD FOR REAL PEOPLE

The USDA's Food Guide Pyramid is one of the most widely recognized nutrition education tools ever used in this country. Unfortunately, *recognizing* this graphic representation of current nutrition guidelines and actually understanding how to put it into practice are two entirely different matters. In this chapter, you'll learn how to interpret a slight modification of the food pyramid and make it work for your healthy lifestyle.

As researchers uncover more information about nutrition and health agencies discover better ways to disseminate this information to the public, these agencies can and should update their educational approach. In fact, a new edition of the USDA's Food Guide Pyramid is scheduled to be released in 2005. It's important to understand, however, that this doesn't invalidate the traditional food pyramid. Other countries have their own culturally appropriate nutrition education pieces as well, and all these tools are simply a means to encourage people around the world to embrace healthy, balanced eating practices.

What Is a Food Pyramid?

Nutrient and calorie needs vary from person to person depending on age, gender, body size, body composition, level of physical activity, and many other conditions. To understand how best to meet these needs, it's helpful to group foods according to the nutrients they provide. A *food pyramid* (see Figure 5.1) is one way to visualize how each food group contributes to your daily needs. The pyramid provides a range of servings for each group. Individuals with lower calorie needs (women, older adults, sedentary people) can choose the lower number of servings from each food group, whereas those with higher calorie needs (men, teenagers, active people) can select the higher number of servings suggested. In Chapter 3, "Uncover the Natural Eater," you learned about the *why* and *how* of eating; now it's time to focus on the *what*.

The following sections help you understand each food group, why it's important, and how to select the most nutrient-rich foods within each group.

note

The term *serving* is used to help you understand the amounts of foods within each group that provide similar levels of calories and nutrients. This does *not* mean that you must limit yourself to one serving when you eat a particular food. For example, if you eat 1 1/2 cups of cooked spaghetti with dinner, you are getting three servings from the grain and starch group (because one serving is one-half cup of cooked pasta). If your calorie needs are on the low end, that's about half your daily needs from this particular food group.

FIGURE 5.1

A food pyramid helps you visualize how to meet your daily nutrient needs.

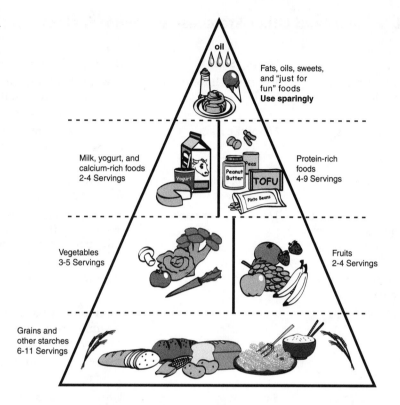

Great Grains and Other Starches

Breads, cereals, pasta, rice, grain products, and starchy vegetables such as potatoes and corn provide complex carbohydrates, B vitamins, iron, fiber, some protein, and many other nutrients. They are generally low in fat and have about 80 to 100 calories per serving. As you learned in Chapter 4, "Balanced Nutrition," try to choose grain products made with whole grains rather than highly processed grains. Starchy vegetables are included with this group because they have a nutrient profile similar to grain foods. If you are sedentary, you may require six or fewer servings from this group daily, whereas highly active people and growing teenagers may need more than 11 servings daily! Table 5.1 provides detailed information about foods included in this group, their serving sizes, and serving tips.

TABLE 5.1 Grains and Other Starches—Premium Fuel for Your Body and Mind!

Food	Serving Size	Healthy Additions
Whole-grain breads, rolls, tortillas	1 slice/small roll/6-inch tortilla	Low-fat or fat-free spreads, jams, lean meat, peanut butter, sliced veggies, cooked beans
Whole-grain pitas, bagels, English muffins, buns	1/2 of the item	Low-fat or fat-free cream cheese, jams, peanut butter, scrambled eggs
Whole-grain cereals	1/2 cup cooked or 1 oz. ready-to-eat cereal	Skim milk, soymilk, raisins, fresh fruit, cinnamon, yogurt
Brown rice, whole-wheat pasta, quinoa, couscous, buckwheat, millet, and other grains	1/3 to 1/2 cup cooked	Marinara sauce, cooked veggies, dried fruits, firm tofu, cooked beans, lean meat/poultry/fish
Whole-grain crackers and rice cakes	3 to 6 of the item	Hummus, low-fat cheese, nut butters
Baked tortilla chips	1 oz.	Salsa, cooked beans, light sour cream, shredded cheddar, cooked chicken
Pretzels	1 oz.	Yogurt dip, mustard, light ranch dressing
Light or air-popped popcorn	3 cups popped	Parmesan cheese, chili powder, garlic powder
Whole-grain pancakes, waffles	One 4-inch item	Fresh chopped fruit, yogurt, light syrup, peanut or soynut butter
Cooked corn, peas, potato, sweet potato	1/2 cup	Cooked beans, salsa, plain yogurt, cinnamon, shredded cheese
Homemade muffins	One small	Tub margarine or nut butters or nothing at all!

Here are some ideas to help you make the most of your grains and starches:

- Most of us use wheat products to the exclusion of other nutritious starchy foods. Use rice, oats, and corn, or try quinoa, millet, and other uncommon grains.

- Mix whole-grain cereal with yogurt and fruit for a meal or a snack.

- Fill soft whole-wheat tortillas with beans, vegetables, lean meats, low-fat cheese, and salsa.

- Eat fewer baked goods with added fats (doughnuts, cakes, cookies, biscuits, croissants).

- Cook old-fashioned rolled oats in large batches—oatmeal keeps well, covered in the refrigerator, for several days.

- Stuff a whole-wheat pita with lean meats, chopped veggies, and a bit of low-fat dressing for a brown bag lunch.

- Add barley to soups and stews for a healthy dose of soluble fiber.

- Flavor cooked rice, couscous, and quinoa with toasted slivered almonds, dried fruit, chopped green onions, fat-free chicken broth, shredded carrots, or leftover cooked vegetables.

- Bake a potato in the microwave by piercing the skin several times with a fork and baking approximately 3–5 minutes (oven times vary). Let sit for a few minutes to continue cooking; then stuff with leftover chili, shredded chicken, tuna salad, cooked broccoli or spinach, low-fat cottage cheese, or salsa.

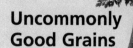

Uncommonly Good Grains

Quinoa is a small round grain that cooks very quickly and is higher in protein than most other grains. It originated in South America, and its mild flavor makes it versatile at the table. Serve it instead of rice or couscous and flavor with chopped, cooked onions, celery, carrots, and spices.

Millet, a little round yellow grain, can be used as a side dish instead of rice or pasta. For a tasty alternative to oatmeal, serve it hot with chopped fruit, nuts, and milk or soymilk.

Vital Vegetables

Vegetables add color and texture to your meals, and vitamins, minerals, antioxidants, phytochemicals, and fiber to your overall diet.

WHAT ARE ANTIOXIDANTS AND PHYTOCHEMICALS?

Antioxidants roam around the body neutralizing destructive substances called free radicals. *Free radicals* are formed both as a result of normal metabolic processes and exposure to toxins in the environment (tobacco, alcohol, pollution, sun exposure, and so on) and have been implicated in heart disease, cancer, and other chronic illnesses. Antioxidants help prevent those free radicals from doing too much damage to body cells and tissues—an extremely important job!

Phytochemicals are substances found only in plants that may have numerous health benefits. Researchers are exploring their role in preventing cancer, heart disease, diabetes, osteoporosis, and many other chronic illnesses.

Include a variety of colorful vegetables to obtain adequate amounts of beta-carotene, vitamin C, iron, potassium, and calcium. Nonstarchy vegetables such as broccoli, cauliflower, tomatoes, peppers, mushrooms, and greens average about 25 calories per serving. At minimum, aim for three servings from this group every day and work your way up to five or more for optimum health! It's not as difficult as you think to get three servings of vegetables when you consider serving size. For example, if you had a cup of salad at lunch (one serving) and a cup of steamed broccoli (two servings) with dinner, you've already met your daily quota. See Table 5.2 for more serving recommendations for vegetables.

TABLE 5.2 Vary Your Vegetable Choices to Maximize Your Nutrient Intake

Food	Serving Size	Healthy Hints
Dark green vegetables (kale; collard, turnip, and mustard greens; spinach)	1 cup raw or 1/2 cup cooked	Top with low-fat salad dressings, a drizzle of olive oil, spices and herbs, lemon zest, and vinegar.
Deep yellow vegetables (carrots, sweet potatoes, pumpkin, winter squash)	1 cup raw or 1/2 cup cooked	Season with nutmeg, ginger, cinnamon, or parsley.
Cruciferous vegetables (broccoli, cauliflower, cabbage, bok choy)	1 cup raw or 1/2 cup cooked	Top with low-fat cheeses, parmesan cheese, lemon pepper, vinegar, mustard, soy sauce, or light dressing.
Others (peppers, mushrooms, zucchini, green beans, leeks, onions, pea pods, tomatoes, cucumber, and so on)	1 cup raw or 1/2 cup cooked	Dip in light ranch dressing, sauté in a little olive oil and garlic, or tuck into sandwiches, tortillas, and pitas.
Low-sodium tomato or vegetable juice	4 to 6 oz.	Serve with a twist of lemon or lime over ice for a summertime cocktail.

These tips can help you incorporate vegetables painlessly:

- Raw vegetables make great snacks—be sure to place them at eye level in the front of the refrigerator for all to see.
- Stock up on frozen and canned vegetables for later in the week; rinse canned varieties under cold running water to reduce the sodium.
- Add chopped vegetables to pasta dishes, soups, sauces, pizza, and casseroles.
- Try quick cooking techniques such as steaming, grilling, stir frying, and microwaving.

- Stock up on prewashed, prediced vegetables from the salad bar to minimize preparation time for recipes.
- Seal chopped onions in premeasured amounts in freezer bags for recipes (double bagging can help prevent other foods from absorbing the onion smell).
- Throw deli-roast chicken on a bed of romaine lettuce; add chopped olives, Parmesan cheese, and low-fat Italian dressing for a quick Caesar salad.
- Scramble eggs or egg substitutes with leftover chopped vegetables and serve with toast and juice for breakfast.
- Top a pita round with spaghetti sauce and leftover chopped veggies and a bit of shredded cheese; broil till crisp and enjoy!

Fabulous Fruits

Fruits are rich in vitamin C, beta-carotene, folic acid, potassium, and fiber, and they add sweetness, color, flavor, and texture to your meals and snacks. They are naturally low in fat and have about 60 to 80 calories per serving. Aim for two to four servings of fruit per day. Table 5.3 can help you get started.

TABLE 5.3 Fruits Add a Flavor Sensation to Meals and Snacks

Food	Serving Size	Healthy Hints
Fresh fruit	1 medium piece (size of tennis ball), 1/2 grapefruit, 1 cup melon, 1/2 to 1 cup berries, 1/2 cup chopped	Citrus fruits (oranges, lemon, grapefruit) and berries are good sources of vitamin C. Deep yellow fruits (apricots, cantaloupe, peaches) are good sources of beta-carotene. Top with cinnamon, nutmeg, chili powder, or plain yogurt with honey.
Canned or frozen fruit	1/2 cup chopped	Choose fruit packed in juice; frozen mixed fruit is a great alternative to fresh—look for no sugar added varieties.
100% fruit juices	4 to 6 oz.	Orange and grapefruit juices are lower in calories and higher in some nutrients than apple, grape, or other juices.
Dried fruits	2 T. to 1/4 cup	Add to hot and cold cereals, cooked rice or couscous, or trail mix or just snack on them plain.

Get your fruit fix with these easy tips:

- Try fruit to satisfy a sweet tooth.

- Enjoy sliced or pureed fruit on pancakes, waffles, cereals, or yogurt.

- Fresh, in-season fruits are the most nutritious and cost-effective choices; bring a bagful to work on Monday morning to last several days.

- Freeze overripe bananas (or use any favorite frozen fruit) and blend with skim or soy milk and a few drops of vanilla extract for a breakfast smoothie.

- Add bits of dried fruit to hot cereals.

- Add drained, canned pineapple to stir fry.

- Have a sliced apple with peanut butter for a midmorning or afternoon snack.

- Serve fresh melon with cottage cheese or yogurt for breakfast. Sprinkle with cinnamon.

- Warm blueberries (fresh or frozen) in the microwave and use to top pancakes, waffles, and French toast.

- Fix a breakfast sandwich to go—spread peanut or soynut butter on whole-wheat bread, toast, or waffles and top with sliced bananas, pears, apples, or strawberries instead of jam.

Marvelous Milk and More than Acceptable Alternatives

Low-fat dairy milk and yogurt and many plant-based dairy alternatives are the best dietary sources of calcium and vitamin D, both of which are associated with positive bone health. Researchers are also examining calcium and other nutrients in milk and yogurt for their capability to promote healthy blood pressure and body weight. These foods are rich in protein, riboflavin, thiamin, and vitamin B12, and vary from 90 to 200 calories per serving due to differences in fat, saturated fat, cholesterol, and sugar content. If you don't drink dairy milk, look for fortified soy or rice milk to meet your calcium and vitamin D needs. Shoot for at least two full 8-ounce servings daily (see Table 5.4 for more information on servings); three or four servings are best for growing teens, pregnant and lactating women, and adults over the age of 50.

TABLE 5.4 Milk, Yogurt, and Alternatives Keep Your Body and Bones in Top Condition

Food	Serving Size	Healthy Hints
Low-fat or skim milk and buttermilk	8 oz.	Choose skim or 1% to reduce fat and saturated fat.
Fortified soy milk	8 oz.	Use plain varieties in place of dairy milk in recipes; try vanilla flavored on cereal and in smoothies; chocolate soymilk makes a delicious sweet treat.
Yogurt, soy yogurt	8 oz.	Choose low-fat, fat-free, and reduced calorie versions.
Nonfat dry milk powder	1/3 cup	Keep a container on hand for emergencies; add to smoothies and hot cereal.
Evaporated skim milk	4 oz.	Use instead of cream in coffee, soups, and recipes.

Here are some ideas to get you back in the milk and yogurt habit:

- Substitute skim or soymilk for water when preparing hot cereals.
- Replace some of the fat in recipes with plain yogurt or buttermilk.
- Add vanilla, lemon, cinnamon, honey, or other flavorings to plain or vanilla yogurt to make a dip for fruits.
- Try fortified soymilk or Lactaid milk if you are lactose sensitive.
- Grab 8-ounce drinkable yogurts for a calcium boost on the go.
- Make your own "cream cheese"—drain the liquid from plain yogurt by placing it in a coffee filter-lined colander over a bowl. Store in the refrigerator for four hours to overnight—the longer it sits, the thicker the consistency. Use instead of sour cream or cream cheese in some recipes or on bagels or baked potatoes.

Protein Packs a Punch

This is the most diverse of any of the food groups and includes lean meats, poultry, fish, and game; cooked legumes; low-fat cheeses; eggs and egg substitutes; soy products; and peanut and soynut butter. It's helpful to think of your daily protein needs in terms of ounces instead of servings or portions because you have such a wide variety of options. Meat, poultry, fish, game, and eggs are good sources of protein,

B vitamins, iron, and zinc. Calories for these foods range from 35 to 100 per ounce, depending on their fat content, and each serving listed in Table 5.5 contains about 7 grams of protein. Low-fat cheeses, though derived from milk, are similar to lean meats in terms of their carbohydrate, fat, and protein content, so they're also included in the protein group. Cooked legumes and soy products are excellent low-fat, carbohydrate-rich sources of protein, whereas peanut and soynut butters (though higher in calories than other choices) are convenient, quick, and rich in heart healthy fats. Most adults need a total of 5 to 9 ounces of protein foods daily, but check with a registered dietitian to determine more specific requirements based on your lifestyle and health history.

TABLE 5.5 Protein Is Abundant in a Wide Variety of Foods

Food	Serving Size	Healthy Hints
Lean beef, veal, pork, lamb	1 oz.	Trim visible fats and use as a complement to your meals rather than as the main course.
Skinless chicken or turkey	1 oz.	Cook in large batches and freeze in individual portions for quick meals all week long.
Fish, tuna, shellfish	1 oz.	It's easy to overcook fish; cook just until opaque throughout and flaking on the edges; combine canned tuna and salmon with a little dressing and stuff into pita rounds or serve on toasted English muffins.
Eggs and egg substitutes	1 large egg or 1/4 cup	Scramble with sautéed vegetables or roll up in a tortilla with cheese and salsa.
Peanut or soynut butter	2 T.	Keep a jar at work to spread on crackers or crunchy fruits for an afternoon snack; use as a spread for toast, pancakes, and waffles instead of butter or stick margarine.
Tofu	4 oz. or 1/2 cup	Use firm varieties in stir-fry or cube and mix with marinara sauce for pasta dishes; add silken varieties to smoothies, dips, and creamy sauces.
Tempeh	1/4 cup	Use instead of ground meats in sloppy Joe recipes, casseroles, and pasta dishes, or grill with barbecue sauce for a sandwich filling or main course.

Food	Serving Size	Healthy Hints
Low-fat cheese, cottage cheese, Parmesan	1 oz., 1/4 cup, and 2 T., respectively	Flavor has improved dramatically in recent years; if you prefer regular versions, simply use a little less to limit fat, saturated fat, and calories.
Soy-based meat alternatives	Varies widely—check labels for serving that provides 7g protein	Soy breakfast sausage, deli meat, hot dogs, burgers, and many other products are convenient meat alternatives; the major drawback is sodium content—one portion often contains more than 400mg of sodium; balance with fresh, unprocessed foods if you use these products.

Make the most of your protein picks with these tips:

- Replace high-fat meats such as bacon, sausage, hot dogs, ribs, and ground beef with lower fat choices such as chicken, turkey, fish, and lean beef or pork.
- Select lean cuts of beef such as eye of round, top round, top sirloin, tenderloin, or flank.
- Most fish and shellfish are very low in fat—choose cod, flounder, haddock, halibut, shrimp, and orange roughy for delicious seafood meals. Fattier fish such as salmon, sardines, mackerel, and tuna are excellent sources of omega-3 fatty acids.
- Add more vegetables, beans, and grains and less meat to soups, stews, casseroles, and entrees.
- Prepare a meatless meal at least once or twice a week; add cooked beans to salad, salsa, potatoes, or pasta; or mash them and use as a sandwich spread or a topping for toast. Experiment with soy-based meat alternatives to burgers, sausage, chicken nuggets, and ground beef—look for them in the frozen food section.
- Sprinkle Parmesan cheese on potatoes, pasta, soup, popcorn, and cooked vegetables.
- Part-skim mozzarella cheese sticks make great snacks with fruit or crackers.
- Most people consume far more animal protein than necessary; use meat as a meal accent rather than as the main course.

Fats, Oils, Sweets, and "Just for Fun" Foods

Fats and oils provide essential fatty acids that your body requires but cannot manufacture on its own. You can obtain essential fatty acids naturally in foods such as fish and some nuts, but pure fats and oils help fill in the gaps. Fats also enhance the flavor of other foods in many dishes. Choose olive, canola, peanut, walnut, flaxseed, and avocado oils rather than butter or stick margarine to emphasize healthier fats. See the section "The Skinny on Fat" in Chapter 4 to refresh your memory about different types of fats and their effects on your overall health. For most people, it is also wise to consider small amounts of nuts and seeds (walnuts, pecans, sunflower seeds, pumpkin seeds, almonds, and many others) part of this group. Although they do provide some protein, most of the calories in nuts and seeds come from heart-healthy fats, so it's best to use them to liven up other dishes rather than as a primary protein source.

Sweets and other "fun foods" can add pleasure and variety to your diet when used in moderation. To enjoy foods from this group without adding excess calories, try the following.

The following suggestions can help you fine-tune your fats and oils:

- Stir-fry vegetables in a bit of olive or canola oil; the fats enable your body to absorb nutrients from the vegetables more efficiently.

- Toss cooked pasta with a little olive oil, fresh basil leaves, salt, pepper, and Parmesan cheese, if desired. Add cooked beans or shrimp for a complete one-pot meal.

- Store chopped walnuts or pecans in the freezer and sprinkle them on hot and cold cereal, yogurt and fruit, spinach salads, and pasta and rice dishes.

- Use sliced avocado rather than mayonnaise on a sandwich or add it to salads for a creamy texture.

- If you're a potato chip aficionado, all the fat-free pretzels in the supermarket won't satisfy your taste for a crispy chip. When you do enjoy these types of foods, be sure to put a helping on a plate instead of eating directly from the bag. It's too easy to eat more than you anticipated when you eat out of the bag!

The following suggestions can help those of you with a sweet tooth to have your cake and eat it too:

- Limit regular soft drinks, "fruit" drinks, and vending machine beverages—they are chock full of calories and essentially devoid of nutrients.

- You needn't cut out candy, cookies, donuts, cakes, and pies completely; simply enjoy them less frequently or in smaller portions. Many people find it helpful to keep only one variety of dessert in their homes—this eliminates the "gotta have a little of everything" syndrome.

■ Use one-fourth less sugar in recipes when you bake at home. Add cinnamon, nutmeg, and cloves to enhance the natural sweetness of baked goods.

■ If you order dessert, split it with several friends—sometimes a few bites of a very rich dessert is all you need to satisfy a sweet tooth.

■ Save your "fun food calories" for the foods you really love—don't settle for six low-fat cookies when what you really crave is a piece of high-quality chocolate.

■ Try adding a dash (or more!) of cinnamon or nutmeg to your coffee grounds before brewing to enhance the taste and cut down on the amount of sugar you add to the finished product.

Try these tips to manage your taste for fun foods:

■ Get enough quality sleep—snack attacks often reflect a lack of energy from poor sleeping habits rather than an addiction to salt and sugar!

■ Include a good source of fiber-rich carbohydrate, lean protein, and a little healthy fat in each main meal to prolong feelings of fullness and satisfaction and cut down on midafternoon munchies.

■ Drink ice water or iced tea with a twist of lemon or lime instead of sugar sweetened beverages.

■ Constant cravings for salty and sweet foods may be an indication that your life could use a boost in the pleasure department; create a list of pleasurable activities in Figure 5.2 that you can employ each day so that you aren't seeking pleasure solely from food.

FIGURE 5.2
Your personal pleasurable activities list.

Read mystery novels
Take a long bath
Go to the driving range
Give yourself a manicure

ALL ABOUT ALCOHOL

Some recent research has shown that moderate alcohol consumption, of red wine in particular, may have long-term health benefits, especially in regards to cardiovascular health. But alcohol consumption is not without risks—even moderate drinking has been associated with an increased risk for breast cancer, and alcohol abuse can wreak havoc on your health, your family, your career, and your life in general. If you have a personal or family history of alcohol addiction or cancer, or you have been diagnosed with diabetes, seek your physician's guidance with respect to alcohol intake.

One alcoholic beverage can contain 95 to 200 calories per serving, so choose wisely and limit yourself to one drink a day or less if you're a woman or two drinks per day or less if you're a man—if you choose to drink at all.

One drink equals

> 5 ounces wine
>
> 12 ounces beer
>
> 1 ounce hard liquor

Making the Most of Your Meals

Until now, you've been learning about your nutrient needs in terms of an entire day's worth of food, but you might still struggle to put individual meals and snacks together. Meal planning is all about balance in flavors, textures, and nutrients. Table 5.6 can help you create satisfying meals that reflect this kind of balance—choose at least one food from each of the three groups at every meal!

Refer to specific food group sections for more details on the types of foods that provide more nutrients for fewer calories.

note

You'll need more than one choice from the fruit/vegetable category at some meals to promote optimal health, but one choice per meal is a great start if you're just getting into the produce habit!

TABLE 5.6   Choose at Least One Food From Each Column at Every Meal

Grains/Starches	Fruit/Vegetable	Protein/Calcium
Ready-to-eat cereals	Bananas, oranges, kiwi	Skim or low-fat dairy milk
Hot cereals, grits	Melon, grapes, apples	Low-fat buttermilk
Bagels	Pears, peaches, nectarines	Fortified soy or rice milk
English muffins	Blueberries, strawberries	Low-fat cheese slices or cubes
Frozen waffles	Blackberries, raspberries	Low-fat cottage cheese
Pancakes	Dried apricots and plums	Low-fat ricotta cheese
Flour/corn tortillas	Raisins or dried cranberries	Low-fat and fat-free yogurt
Bread or toast	Canned or frozen fruits	Soy-based yogurt or cheese
Crackers	Canned or frozen vegetables	Peanut and soynut butter
Rice, quinoa, couscous	100% fruit or vegetable juices	Lean cold cuts
Pasta	Mixed green salads	Eggs and egg substitutes
Lentils and cooked beans	Zucchini, squash, tomatoes	Lentils and cooked beans
Barley	Cucumbers, mushrooms	Lean meats, poultry, fish, game
Pita rounds	Kale, spinach, greens	Canned tuna, chicken, salmon
Baked potatoes	Green beans, radishes	Tofu, tempeh
Popcorn	Cabbage, Brussels sprouts	Soy-based meat alternatives
Cooked corn or polenta	Broccoli, cauliflower, bok choy	
	Tomato or marinara sauce	
	Prepackaged cut vegetables	
	Salsa, fresh or canned	
	Chunky vegetable soups	

The following ideas illustrate how you might assemble quick, tasty meals using foods from Table 5.6.

Breakfast

Many clients complain that eating breakfast starts a vicious cycle of getting hungry at regular intervals for the rest of the day. Guess what? That's great! It means that your metabolism is working properly and your body's signals are reflecting that. If you don't enjoy typical breakfast foods, try sandwiches, pizza, or other lunch and dinner items instead. The following breakfast ideas are quick, easy, and taste good, so no more excuses!

- Top whole-grain cereal with skim or soymilk, chopped walnuts, and sliced banana.

- Scramble eggs or egg substitute with chopped onions, peppers, and broccoli; sprinkle with cheese and wrap in a warm whole-wheat tortilla.

- Top an English muffin with spaghetti sauce and low-fat cheese and broil; serve with a glass of orange juice.

- Fill half a small cantaloupe with yogurt or cottage cheese and sprinkle with low-fat granola.

- Top toasted frozen waffles with peanut butter or ricotta cheese and frozen raspberries that have been warmed in the microwave.

- Make old-fashioned oatmeal with skim or soymilk in the microwave and top with chopped pecans and dried cranberries.

- Spread whole-grain toast, a bagel, or an English muffin with peanut butter and serve with milk and fruit.

- Heat cooked rice with skim milk or soymilk and chopped dried fruits.

Lunch or Dinner

If you struggle with lunch and dinner choices, you might need to restock your cabinets at home and work so that you have the ingredients for "throw-together" meals. These meals don't need to be elaborate to be satisfying and nutritious. Try some of the following super-fast lunch and dinner options the next time you're contemplating takeout.

- Heat your choice of rinsed, canned beans with salsa and cheese and roll up in a whole-grain tortilla.

- Stir-fry chicken breast strips or firm tofu cubes and frozen vegetables in olive oil and serve over brown minute rice.

- Toss cooked, whole-wheat pasta with canned tomatoes, white beans, and fresh spinach; heat through and enjoy.

- Top a baked potato with cottage cheese or plain yogurt and salsa; or warm up a can of vegetarian chili and pour it over the hot potato.

- Microwave precooked polenta rounds with spaghetti sauce and mozzarella cheese.

- Serve a meatless burger on a toasted, whole-grain bun; top with lettuce, tomato, ketchup, and mustard; serve with fresh fruit.

- Stuff a whole-wheat pita with lean ham and Swiss cheese and warm in the microwave. Serve with sliced pears.

- Have breakfast for dinner!

- Add cooked shrimp or chicken breast strips to tossed salad. Top with chopped, toasted pecans and low-fat vinaigrette dressing and serve with crusty bread.

- Add drained, rinsed red kidney beans and salsa to cooked brown rice and heat through.

- Split a pita round and top with spaghetti sauce, fresh or sautéed veggies, and cheese; broil to toast the pita and melt the cheese.

- Use fresh fruit topped with a dollop of vanilla yogurt and a sprinkle of cinnamon for dessert any time!

The Absolute Minimum

So that's it! You should now have a grasp of the types of foods that meet your body's needs for nutrients and your taste buds' needs for flavor.

- A food pyramid helps you visualize how each main food group contributes to your daily diet.

- Look beyond the graphic—get to know serving sizes to apply food pyramid recommendations.

- Try to include at least three food groups in your meals to get the nutrients you need and stay satisfied longer.

- Make changes slowly; pick and choose a few new food items or recipes each week to avoid feeling too overwhelmed.

IN THIS CHAPTER

- Read food labels consistently and confidently
- Understand why it pays to be skeptical about claims made on packaging
- Make the most of your time, money, and nutrition knowledge at the grocery store

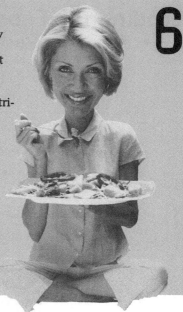

6

THE SAVVY SHOPPER

Confusion about nutrition information is at an all-time high. Consumers are increasingly pressed for time and energy and are looking to maximize their grocery dollar. Studies are released daily that seem to contradict what you know (or thought you knew) about good, common sense nutrition. Eggs are bad; eggs might lower cholesterol. Butter is heart disease in a stick; margarine is one step away from plastic. Eat more fresh produce; outbreaks of food-borne illnesses are linked to some fruits and vegetables. It's no wonder consumers are tired, frustrated, and ready to throw in the towel when it comes to making informed decisions about what to eat! This chapter clears up the confusion and provides a framework on which to base your food-buying decisions. You'll start by getting a grasp on the information on the food labels themselves, and then move on to aisle-specific guidance in the grocery store. Your goal isn't to become a card-carrying member of the "food police," only to increase your awareness of what you choose to put in your body.

Decoding the Food Label

Reading food labels helps you learn about food products, their ingredients, and their nutritional values, and is a key skill in choosing healthy foods. The standards for food labels in the United States fall under the direction of the Food and Drug Administration's Center for Food Safety and Applied Nutrition (CFSAN). Stay abreast of changes to food label information and legislation by checking out CFSAN's website on food labeling and nutrition at www.cfsan.fda.gov/~dms/lab-gen.html.

The information found on food packaging falls into four main categories:

- Nutrition Facts panel
- Ingredient list
- Health claims
- Nutrient content claims

We'll cover each category of information in detail. You might find it helpful to choose one or two key areas to examine on food labels each week, as opposed to trying to remember all of it the next time you hit the aisles. Take your time and remember that *all* foods can fit into a healthy diet!

Getting All the Facts—The Nutrition Facts Panel

With slick packaging and descriptions, manufacturers can make nearly anything look good on the grocery store shelves, but the *Nutrition Facts panel* is *the* place to go for the most straightforward information found on the entire label. This treasure trove of data is usually on the side or back of the package and is designed to give you an idea of how the product contributes to your total daily nutrient needs. Refer to Figure 6.1 while you're learning about each of these sections.

Start with Serving Size Information

Every value on the Nutrition Facts panel is based on the nutrients found in *one* serving, so if you look at nothing else on the label, pay attention to this section! Most people are surprised at how small the serving sizes on packages seem compared to the amounts they typically consume. Many beverages, for example, are sold in 16- or 20-ounce bottles, but list the serving size as only 8 ounces. If you drink the whole bottle, you'll be getting two or more times the amount of nutrients indicated on the Nutrition Facts panel!

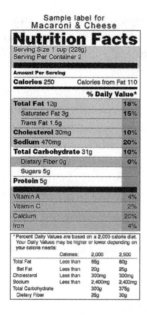

FIGURE 6.1

Understanding the Nutrition Facts panel. (Source: www.cfsan.fda. gov/~dms/ foodlab.html)

Calories and Calories from Fat

This line follows the serving size information and tells you how many calories each serving provides and how many of those calories come from fat. The calories from fat are calculated by multiplying the total grams of fat per serving by nine (because each gram of fat contains nine calories):

Calories from fat = total grams of fat per serving × 9 calories per gram

Don't pigeonhole products based on their calories from fat; some nutritious foods (nuts or avocados, for example) get a majority of their calories from fat, whereas many not-so-nutritious foods (such as low-fat cookies and snack chips) get only a small percentage of their total calories from fat.

Nutrients and % Daily Values

Now you're moving on to specific nutrients. Total fat, saturated fat, cholesterol, sodium, total carbohydrates (fiber and sugar), protein, vitamins A and C, calcium, and iron are the nutrients included on most labels. Some may also include mono- and polyunsaturated fats and fortified vitamins and minerals. Information about these nutrients can appear in one or both of the following forms:

- In terms of the amount by weight per serving (examples: 3g of fat, 300mg of sodium)
- As a percentage (%) of the daily value for a 2,000 calorie reference diet (example: 12% of the daily value for dietary fiber)

Some Nutrition Facts panels on larger packages add a footnote that provides more detail on this reference diet used to calculate the % Daily Values. This particular diet may or may not be appropriate for you personally, but it does provide a standard way of drawing comparisons among products.

By using the % Daily Values, you can easily determine how a particular food contributes to your total daily nutrient needs. Compare different brands of similar products to determine which contain higher percentages for nutrients you want to emphasize, such as fiber or calcium. Look to see whether the nutrients you want to limit, such as saturated fat and sodium, have lower percentages. For example, if you have recently been diagnosed with hypertension (high blood pressure), you need to pay attention to the level of sodium in foods you use frequently. If you're shopping for spaghetti sauce and one jar lists 15% as the % Daily Value for sodium, and the other lists 25%, which would you choose? If both seem equally appealing in terms of taste, the brand that contains only 15% of your daily sodium intake would better meet your particular needs.

Ingredient List—What's In *Your* Food?

A list of ingredients appears on almost all food products and can be an important source of information for cultural, allergy, and general health reasons. The ingredients are listed in decreasing order by weight, so the first ingredients are present in much higher amounts than the last ingredients. In general, look for products with shorter ingredient lists. Are there healthy foods out there with lots of ingredients? Sure, but as a rule, the longer the list, the more processed the food.

Health Claims

Health claims are statements on packages that describe the relationship between a nutrient and a disease or health-related condition. This particular area of the food label has gone through some major changes in the last several years because consumers are clamoring for more information about the foods they eat and how those foods might be contributing to their health and well being. Under current law, there are three major categories of health claims, so put on your thinking cap and prepare yourself for some hard-core label lingo.

Health Claims That Meet Significant Scientific Agreement (a.k.a. the Most Reliable Claims)

These are top-notch claims that have stood the test of time and scientific scrutiny. Note that these claims state that there is a strong *relationship* between a food or food substance and a disease or health-related condition, *not* that the food or nutrient can *prevent, treat, or cure* the condition. Table 6.1 summarizes these claims.

TABLE 6.1   Health Claims That Meet Significant Scientific Agreement

Diets...	Reduce the risk of...
High in calcium	Osteoporosis
Low in total fat	Cancer
Low in saturated fat and cholesterol	Coronary heart disease
High in fiber-containing grain products, fruits, and vegetables	Cancer
High in fruits and vegetables	Cancer
High in fruits, vegetables, and grain products that contain fiber, particularly soluble fiber	Coronary heart disease
High in soluble fiber from certain foods	Coronary heart disease
Lower in sodium	Hypertension
That contain soy protein (25g per day)	Coronary heart disease
That contain plant sterol/stanol esters	Coronary heart disease
With adequate folic acid (400mg per day)	Neural tube defects (affect the brain of a developing fetus)

In addition, packages may state that sugar alcohols do not promote dental caries.

Qualified Health Claims

Now you're entering the gray area of health claims on the food label. *Qualified health claims* are categorized as such because they do not meet the requirements for significant scientific agreement as set forth by the FDA. Manufacturers must petition the FDA to begin using qualified health claims on labels, and when the claims do appear on packaging, a *qualifying* statement (such as "supportive but not conclusive evidence shows that_____") must be included. The next logical question is this: Just how much evidence is required to petition for a claim? That depends. The FDA has not issued a final ruling on qualified claims, but in the interim, three different categories of evidence are provided in the guidelines—*good to moderate level* of scientific agreement; *low level* of scientific agreement; and *very low level* of scientific agreement. At this time, food manufacturers are not likely to submit a petition for a claim for which there is a very low level of scientific agreement, but don't buy a product specifically because of a qualified health claim.

Structure/Function Claims

To complicate matters even more, manufacturers are getting around the entire issue by using *structure/function claims*. Structure/function claims draw attention to the relationship between a food or food substance and structures or functions of the human body. This third type of claim is not reviewed by the FDA and is not technically a health claim, but even the savviest consumers find it difficult to tell the difference. For example, some packages contain statements such as "promotes healthy eyes" or "maintains immune function." Although these statements make no reference to a specific disease or health-related condition, they sure sound like it!

The bottom line with all claims is the age-old adage—if it sounds too good to be true, it probably is.

Nutrient Content Claims

Nutrient content claims are (thankfully) fairly cut and dried. These claims are really more like nutrition descriptions and include terms such as *light, free, reduced in*, and so forth. The FDA has set specific guidelines regarding the meaning of these terms, so they can be useful if you understand the definition of the term. Many consumers assume, however, that foods labeled in this manner are necessarily more nutritious or lower in calories than their regular counterparts, and this simply isn't the case. Compare the labels of regular and reduced-fat peanut butter, for example. On closer inspection, you will notice that although the reduced-fat version does have fewer grams of fat, the calorie content per serving is virtually identical to the regular variety. It's always a good idea to look at the Nutrition Facts panel to really understand what you're purchasing. Table 6.2 helps you make sense of some of the most common nutrient content claims.

TABLE 6.2 Nutrient Content Claims—Know What You're Getting!

What the Label Says	What It Means
Low fat	3g or less per serving
Low sodium	140mg or less per serving
Low cholesterol	20mg or less per serving
Cholesterol free	Less than 2mg cholesterol and 2g or less of saturated fat per serving
Low calorie	40 calories or less per serving
Lean	Less than 10g fat, 4.5g or less saturated fat, and less than 95mg cholesterol per 100g
Extra lean	Less than 5g fat, less than 2g saturated fat, and less than 95mg cholesterol per 100g

What the Label Says	What It Means
Reduced	At least 25% less of a nutrient or calories than the regular product
Light or lite	1/3 fewer *calories* than a standard product or
	More than 50% less *fat* than a standard product or
	More than 50% less *sodium* than a standard product or
	May refer to the texture or color (as in "light brown sugar")
% fat free	Reflects the amount of fat in 100 grams of the food
Dietetic	One or more ingredients has been changed, substituted, or restricted
Sugar free or sugarless	Less than 0.5g sugars per serving and contains no ingredients that are sugars or that contain sugars; not necessarily low calorie
Very low sodium	35mg or less sodium per serving
Sodium free	Less than 5mg of sodium per serving
Fat free	Less than 0.5g of fat per serving and no added fat or oil
Good source of fiber	2.5 to 4.9g per serving
High fiber	5g or more per serving

Smart Shopping Tips

Now it's time to put your label-reading knowledge to good use! Meal planning and regular grocery shopping are essential in developing your healthy lifestyle. If your refrigerator, freezer, and pantry are stocked with healthy foods, you are more likely to eat a well-balanced diet. Learning to make the most economical and nutritious selections in the grocery store may be challenging at first, but the following tips will help you shop smarter and healthier:

- Shop from a list.
  - A flexible grocery list ensures that you select the foods you need, decreases temptations to buy foods displayed throughout the store, and can save time and money.
  - Start with weekly specials and build your menu and subsequent list from those items.
  - Keep your list in a prominent place so that all members of the household can contribute.
  - Use the information in the section "Navigating Miles of Aisles" later in this chapter to help devise your list.

- Allow adequate time for shopping.
  - Plan to shop when you have extra time to read food labels and compare your typical picks with healthier fare (at least in the beginning). You won't need to do this every time, but the initial investment will pay off.
  - Shop when the store is less crowded so that you can be more relaxed and have extra space and time; try early morning, late at night, and weekdays instead of weekends.
- Shop on a satisfied stomach. Shopping while you are hungry makes you vulnerable to convenience foods and anything on special. Don't do it to yourself!
- Start in the produce department.
  - If you fill your cart with nutritious foods first, you'll have less room for packaged and processed foods!
  - Plan for extra time when you get home for washing and chopping fresh vegetables so that they're ready for recipes later in the week. This minimizes the "rotting cauliflower syndrome."
- Use coupons cautiously. Use coupons only for items that you need and compare unit prices for the best deals. Many times, purchasing name brand products with coupons is still more expensive than store brands.

Navigating Miles of Aisles

The following information is designed to help you navigate each section of the grocery store successfully and provide some tips for food preparation after you get the groceries to your kitchen. These are merely *suggestions*! Feel free to modify them to meet your needs and preferences.

Produce Department and Juices

Nothing beats fresh, locally grown produce from a farmer's market, but let's face it; very little of the produce we consume is actually grown close to home. Some stores offer virtually hundreds of choices from growers around the world. It's easy to get carried away, but keep this rule of thumb in mind when shopping for fresh produce: Purchase only as much as you can reasonably consume within four to five days. The longer fruits and vegetables sit in the crisper drawer, the greater the nutrient loss. (There are a few exceptions; apples and citrus fruits keep well in the refrigerator for several weeks, for example.) Shop again in the middle of the week for a few more fruits and vegetables, or rely on frozen and canned produce until your next trip to the store. Here are some additional tips:

- Convenience/precut items may be more expensive but are worth every penny if they enable you to increase your fruit and vegetable intake. Try getting recipe-ready vegetables right off the salad bar!

- Lettuce and leafy greens—the darker, the more nutrient rich (that is, romaine, endive, kale, and spinach contain more nutrients than iceberg lettuce).

- Prepared salads are convenient and may decrease waste. Check the expiration date and look for fresh, crisp greens with no sign of wilting or discoloration. Be sure to wash them (even if they say "triple washed") before digging in—increasing numbers of people are getting sick due to bacterial contamination of packaged produce.

- Enjoy seasonal fruits and vegetables and try different varieties of the same item. If you love fresh berries, purchase them on sale and freeze on cookie sheets for use later in the year.

- Fruit juice versus fruit drinks—fresh fruit is best in terms of fiber, vitamins, and minerals, but 100% fruit juice can help you meet your nutrient needs, too. Try calcium and vitamin D fortified juices if you find it difficult to get the recommended number of daily dairy servings. Fruit drinks contain little in the way of real juice or nutrition and should be an infrequent choice.

- Potatoes—Try red, sweet, or new potatoes. Top baked or microwaved potatoes with salsa, plain yogurt, low-fat cheese, cooked vegetables, chili, spicy beans, or cottage cheese.

- Remember: Wash, chop, and place prepared vegetables in airtight bags right when you get home from the store!

Meat, Poultry, and Seafood Section

We just love our animal proteins, don't we? The following suggestions can help you enjoy your favorites without going overboard on saturated fats and calories:

- Choose high-fat meats such as sausage, ribs, bacon, and hamburger less frequently.

- Look for lean cuts of red meat such as *round*, *sirloin*, *top loin*, and *flank* cuts.

- Highly marbled meats come with a hefty calorie, fat, and saturated fat price—use sparingly!

- Higher fat meats can be prepared with dry heat methods (bake, broil, or grill), whereas lean meats taste better with slow, moist cooking methods (baste, braise, marinate, or stew).

- Ground turkey with skin contains almost as much fat as regular ground beef. Ask your butcher for ground turkey breast without skin.

- When choosing poultry, dark meat is slightly higher in fat but also contains more iron. Remove the skin to save significant calories, cholesterol, and saturated fat. Cook all types of poultry in large batches and freeze in individual portions for quick meals.

- Deli meats are convenient, but most are high in sodium, and some can be high in fat as well. Ask for nutrition information and try to use fresh meats more often.

- Check labels on special products—turkey bologna, franks, and bacon may be just as high in fat and calories as their regular counterparts.

- Fresh seafood shouldn't smell "fishy"; if it does, shop elsewhere or stick to frozen.

- If you're new to eating fish, try mild varieties such as tilapia, orange roughy, and other whitefish before tackling more strongly flavored varieties such as salmon.

Dairy Case

"Dairy case" is a bit of a misnomer with all the plant-based alternatives available today. If you choose to meet your calcium needs with true dairy products, look for reduced-fat versions of your favorites. This is one area in which low-fat products do provide significant health advantages over full-fat counterparts. As always, you are free to make your own choices about reduced-fat products; some people enjoy skim milk, and others think it tastes like water. It might be in your best interest to use 1% or 2% milk and reduce your intake of saturated fat elsewhere in your diet. The following concepts can help you make your "dairy decisions":

- Notice label and nutritional content differences between skim, 1%, 2%, and whole milk. Calcium content is almost identical, but fat, calories, and saturated fat vary greatly.

- Plain yogurt is great to use in place of mayonnaise, sour cream, or salad dressing in various recipes. An 8-ounce carton of sugar-sweetened (even if low-fat or fat-free) yogurt can contain more than 200 calories. If you consume yogurt frequently, you might consider sweetening plain yogurt yourself with fresh fruit or a little honey—you'll probably use far less than the manufacturer would have.

- For baking purposes, stick butter and margarine are both high in the types of fats that may increase your risk for heart disease; your best bet is to reduce the amount used in the recipe slightly and enjoy rich foods and desserts in smaller amounts or less frequently. Soft, tub-style spreads made with olive or canola oils are better choices for topping toast, cooked vegetables, and baked potatoes.

- Diet or reduced calorie margarines have less fat and fewer calories than regular margarine, but most cannot be used for baking.

- Try reduced-fat cheese products; quality has improved greatly! If you don't like the taste or texture of these products, try mixing a little regular cheese in with them, or resolve to make cheese an occasional treat and use the real stuff in smaller quantities.

- Experiment with soy milk, yogurt, and cheese; many fortified soy products are excellent sources of heart-healthy soy protein, calcium, vitamin D, and B vitamins. These products are great alternatives for people who have lactose intolerance or who avoid milk for other reasons.

- Low-fat cottage cheese is an excellent source of protein; try it blended with seasonings for dips; place a scoop on your salad for a heartier meal; mix with applesauce or chopped fruit for breakfast; and use in place of full-fat ricotta cheese in lasagna.

Breads/Bagels/Muffins

In today's carb-phobic culture, it's tempting to purchase reduced-carbohydrate products, or skip this section altogether. Don't bow to peer pressure! Remember, you learned in Chapter 4, "Balanced Nutrition," that carbohydrates are not evil, and they play a vital role in your overall health. These tips can help you get the most nutritional bang for your carbohydrate buck:

- Look for products that list *whole wheat* or *whole grain* as the first ingredient and those that contain more grams of dietary fiber per serving than regular products. Many bread items masquerade as whole-grain products by using words such as *cracked wheat, nine grain, enriched wheat, honey wheat,* and many other healthy-sounding descriptions. Don't be fooled! Refer to Figure 4.1 to refresh your memory about what constitutes a true whole grain.

- Choose English muffins, toast, or small frozen bagels more often than fresh bagels and save from 100 to 200 calories per serving!

- Muffins in the bakery department are loaded with sugar, fat, and calories. One muffin may contain more than 20 grams of fat and 300 calories. Consider making healthier muffins at home in large batches and freezing for quick breakfasts and snacks.

- Try whole-wheat pitas and tortillas for meals on the go; stuff with lean deli meats, fresh spinach, chopped veggies, and a bit of vinaigrette dressing for lunch; fruit and peanut butter go great in a breakfast pita; or scramble eggs and roll up in a tortilla with salsa any time of day…delicious!

Canned Foods

Food snobs take note—canned produce actually retains more nutrients than fresh produce that has been trucked across the country, sat in the display case for a couple days, and stored in your refrigerator for a week before you finally get around to eating it. Yes, there may be a flavor and texture difference, but many people are willing to sacrifice a little in those areas for the convenience canned foods offer. You know yourself best—use these tips to improve the nutrition profile of your canned food choices:

- Canned fruits packed in their own juice or light syrup have less added sugar and fewer calories than canned fruit packed in heavy syrup. It isn't much of an issue either way if you don't drink the juice or syrup!

- Canned vegetables are similar in nutrition content to fresh vegetables (and sometimes better) but usually contain more sodium. Put canned vegetables in a strainer and rinse with cold water to reduce the sodium or buy *no added salt* varieties.

- Canned soups and tomato products (pastes, sauces) are generally very high in sodium. Look for low sodium or *no added salt* varieties. Cream soups can be high in fat; look for reduced fat varieties.

- Canned beans are great to keep on hand to pump up soups, salads, spaghetti sauce, pasta and rice dishes, and more. They're more convenient than dried beans, but are also (you guessed it) higher in sodium. Check the labels for lower sodium products. As with canned vegetables, you can greatly reduce the sodium content by draining and rinsing under cold water.

Frozen Foods

As we spend less time preparing our own meals, we spend more of our food budget on prepared frozen foods. Label-reading skills come in handy in this department because nutrition content varies so widely among products. Here are some hints to help you navigate the frozen food section:

- Frozen fruits and vegetables are convenient and generally as nutritious as fresh produce. Use frozen fruit in breakfast smoothies with milk or soymilk, yogurt, and/or juice. Throw cooked frozen vegetables in with macaroni and cheese, couscous, or marinara sauce.

- In frozen meals, calorie, sodium, and fat content varies greatly. Compare labels! Some "healthy" frozen meals do not provide enough calories for active individuals—supplement with fruit, salad, and yogurt. Balance out your day with fresh, low-sodium meals and snacks.

- Frozen chicken, fish, and shrimp can be a convenient alternative to fresh. Follow package instructions for thawing and avoid thawing any food at room temperature.

- Soy-based meat alternatives abound in the frozen food section. Try soy breakfast sausages, burgers, chicken patties, chicken nuggets, and ground beef crumbles. Most can be fully cooked in the microwave in less than two minutes.

- Some frozen yogurts and light ice creams contain less fat and saturated fat than regular ice cream but similar calorie contents; will you be tempted to have two scoops of a low-fat frozen treat simply because it's "healthier"? Be sure to read labels and enjoy any type of dessert in moderation!

Condiments, Baking, and Spices

The following items improve the flavor and nutrition content of everyday dishes:

- Purchase a variety of spices and herbs to enhance the flavor of foods and reduce sodium in recipes. Seasoning blends are especially nice for beginner cooks and people looking to streamline the food preparation process. Store all spices and herbs in a cool, dry place (preferably far from the stove and oven!).

- Keep nonstick pans and cooking spray available for quick, nutritious meal preparation.

- Canola oil is a good choice for baking because it is flavorless. Olive oil is ideal for salad dressings and as a dip for bread and rolls. Both types are mainly monounsaturated fats. Peanut, walnut, flaxseed (linseed), avocado, and many other gourmet oils can add pizzazz to your dishes—use all oils in moderate amounts.

- Mustard, ketchup, low-sodium soy sauce, marinades, salsa, olives, pesto, and light salad dressings are flavorful additions—monitor the amount to keep sodium in check.

- Lemons, limes, flavored vinegars, and bottled minced garlic and ginger are high-flavor, low-calorie choices—use liberally in your favorite dishes!

- Purchase 100% whole-wheat flour for your baking needs—you can substitute it for part of the all-purpose flour in many recipes. Whole-wheat *pastry* flour can be used instead of all-purpose flour in most recipes and provides a light texture with whole-wheat goodness.

- Look for whole-wheat pancake and waffle mixes—great alternatives to regular quick baking mixes!

■ Find ground flaxseed meal in the specialty flour section of many grocery stores. Store it in the freezer or refrigerator to keep those healthy omega-3 fatty acids fresh longer. Sprinkle on cold or hot cereal or toast, stir into yogurt, or use for part of the fat in homemade baked goods.

■ Keep nonfat dry milk powder on hand to boost calcium in soups, stews, hot cereal, and smoothies (also comes in handy for "end of the week" milk needs!).

■ Keep a bag of chopped nuts (almonds, walnuts, pecans, and so on) in the freezer for adding to salads, cereals, baked goods, yogurt, homemade trail mix, and even for coating fish and chicken before baking!

Snacks

Snacks can help you manage your appetite so that you arrive at the next meal hungry but not starving. If it will be more than an hour or two before your next meal, include a source of carbohydrate (from fruit, crackers, pretzels, and so on) and a little protein (from milk, cheese, yogurt, lean meat, peanut butter, or nuts) for more staying power. Here are some ideas to get you out of your current snack rut:

■ Look for baked chips and pretzels rather than potato chips, cheese puffs, and tortilla chips. Or make your own chips by cutting tortillas or pitas into wedges and baking till crisp. Add nonstick spray and spices as desired. Light microwave and air-popped popcorn are good sources of fiber.

■ Sweet snacks such as graham crackers, fig cookies, vanilla wafers, and animal crackers make lower fat choices than cookies, donuts, and cakes, but remember that these items still contain fair amounts of calories, so be smart with serving sizes.

■ Dried fruits are high in fiber, nutrients, and calories. Use them in small amounts in cooked cereals and to make your own trail mix with dry cereal, almonds, peanuts, pretzels, and so on.

■ Look for no-salt or lightly salted nuts and nut mixes.

■ Some of the best snacks are mini-meals. Try yogurt with granola or chopped nuts, a small bowl of whole-grain cereal with milk, a banana or an apple with a tablespoon of peanut butter, whole-wheat crackers with string cheese or hummus (a spread made from chickpeas), cottage cheese with peaches or pineapple, or toast with sliced cheese and tomato—use your imagination. Snacks don't have to come out of a bag!

Dry Staples/Packaged Foods

There are just a few items we've yet to cover, so this group is a catch-all:

- Keep a variety of grains and starchy foods available and look for whole-grain varieties. Noodles, rice, pasta, couscous, bulgur, millet, barley, corn meal, and many other dry staples can form the basis of quick, healthy, balanced meals.

- Limit pasta, noodle, or rice mixes that contain or call for sauces, butter, cheese, or high-sodium seasoning packets. If you use them, experiment with adding only part of the packet's contents to the final dish.

- Dried beans are cheaper than canned, and you can control the amount of added sodium. Cook in large batches and freeze in smaller quantities to add to soups, stews, salads, pasta dishes, salsa, and homemade burritos and tacos. They are a delicious source of complex carbohydrates, protein, and fiber!

- Try evaporated skim milk as a substitute for cream in some recipes or in coffee or tea.

- Peanut butter is a great all-purpose ingredient in quick, grab-and-go meals and snacks. Try a grilled peanut butter and banana sandwich (an Elvis classic!); add shredded carrots and chopped fruit to a peanut butter sandwich; dip baby carrots or apples in peanut butter that has been warmed to soften; mix a tablespoon into your morning oatmeal. Peanut butter is a great source of heart-healthy monounsaturated fat and provides some protein as well. Be sure to monitor your portions, as the calories can add up quickly!

THE ABSOLUTE MINIMUM

Are you ready to tackle the supermarket and all it entails with your label reading skills? Commit these concepts to memory before you part with your hard-earned money.

- For the most basic, reliable information on the food label, skip the marketing gimmicks on the front of the package and go straight for the Nutrition Facts panel.

- Foods labeled *light*, *reduced in*, or *free*, are not necessarily lower in calories than their regular counterparts.

- Smart shoppers create a flexible grocery list, shop when stores are less crowded, and try to avoid shopping when hungry.

- No single food is going to make or break your eating plan; making consistent, balanced choices over time will!

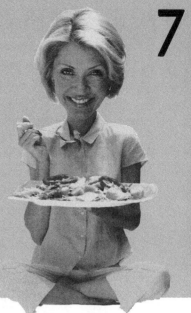

7

Healthy Eating on the Go

When enjoyment and health are priorities, you naturally begin to seek out more variety. Processed foods lose their appeal as you experience the pleasure of fresh foods prepared simply at home. Negative emotions that often surround your eating experiences give way to more positive ones—satisfaction instead of guilt, relaxation instead of haste, and self-awareness instead of restriction. When you make food a priority rather than a nuisance or an obsession, you can rest assured that you are well on your way to a healthier lifestyle.

That said, you still need to be able to make sound choices when dining out. On some hectic nights, your best-laid plans to fix a nutritious meal yourself will simply need to be shelved. For help in choosing meals from fine dining, carryout, and fast food establishments, read on!

The Nature of the Beast

Many countries are known for their particular cuisines and culinary traditions. You might think of sumptuous cheeses, wines, and pastries from France; multiple-course dinners eaten late and leisurely in Italy; and dark ales, hearty sausage, and sauerkraut from Germany.

Each of these countries has its own gastronomic history. In the United States, however, the focus on food has been taken to an entirely different level. We are bombarded by advertisements for fast food, convenience foods, sugar-laden beverages, and heavily fortified foods, all the while hearing messages that this nation is getting heavier, less fit, and more diseased.

The billions of dollars that go into marketing these products have shaped our culture, our food intake, and our health. If your ultimate goal is to create a sustainable, satisfying, and health-promoting lifestyle for you and your family, you need to take a long, hard look at your use of restaurants, fast food, and convenience foods. Can healthy people utilize and even enjoy these conveniences? Absolutely! Do healthy people do this all the time? Probably not.

Eating should be one of life's pleasures and should be a reflection of your personal preferences, cultural background, and overall health. Instead of relegating meals to the back burner, hastily fitting them in when you get a spare moment, make nutrition and taste your priorities; in doing so, you will find that your desire to prepare your own food increases, and your culinary skills will improve with time and practice. Meals as simple as a sandwich and fruit can be immensely more satisfying if you take a moment to relax, set an attractive table, present the food in an appealing way, and share it with others if you have the opportunity. Look at mealtime as a chance not only to nourish your body but your mind and soul as well. This may be a difficult transition to make, but the rewards are great.

After you've made the healthy living commitment, you'll probably be dining out less frequently, but when you do, make choices that honor both your health and your taste buds. The following two sections are particularly pertinent if you eat out more than once or twice a week (and I know there are plenty of you!). We'll start with fast food tips and move on to the S.T.O.P. technique for more leisurely sit-down style meals at restaurants. Those of you who eat out less often can afford a little more latitude when perusing the menu than those who consume a large percentage of their meals outside the home.

Fast Food Follies

Fast food chains have become a dominant force in American culture. They are the largest purchasers of beef, chicken, potatoes, and many other food products. They are found at every highway exit, in every city and town, in many school cafeterias, and in every major airport. In short, fast food places are everywhere.

Although typical fast food fare is high in calories, fat, saturated fat, preservatives, sodium, and added sugars and low in vital nutrients, many establishments are beginning to offer a variety of more nutritious options. It pays to do your homework when it comes to making these healthier options work for your new lifestyle. Most chains offer detailed nutrition information on all products on their websites—look up your usual picks and see whether equally tasty, but more nutritious, items are available. Use the following guidelines to make the best of fast food fare:

- Portion sizes are one of the main culprits of fast food-related weight gain. Order smaller sandwiches and skip the mega-sized value meals—those "great deals" don't do anything for your waistline or your health. Better still, order a sandwich and water or iced tea and bring a piece of fruit from home.

- Choose grilled over crispy or fried sandwiches; the difference could mean 200 calories and 20 grams of fat!

- Skip the mayo, cheese, "special sauce," and regular salad dressings—they add anywhere from 50 to 200 extra calories to your meal. Choose fat-free or reduced-calorie dressings, barbecue sauce, ketchup, mustard, pickles, salsa, and light mayo or sour cream instead.

- Soft drinks and shakes are some of the worst offenders when it comes to excess calories and added sugars. One extra large cola may contain more than 400 calories, and a medium shake can pack more than 700 calories! Choose water, diet colas, unsweetened iced tea, skim milk, or black coffee instead.

- Balance high-fat items with low-fat items. Order a garden salad and reduced-calorie dressing with your sandwich instead of fries.

- Choose English muffins or toast over biscuits, croissants, and hash browns.

- Avoid ordering *double*, *jumbo*, or *super* anything!

- Beware of marketing ploys—menu items marketed to "adult tastes" may still come with hefty amounts of calories and fat.

- Specialty salads are offered at many restaurants, but check out the nutrition facts before you order them in the name of health! Some of these salads have as many calories and as much fat and sodium as the value meals, especially if you add the packets of dressing and "crunchies" that are included. They're a decent way to get your veggies, but don't expect too much from them.

Fine Dining Reminder—S.T.O.P.

It's time to move on to some fine dining skills. To help you make better decisions at sit-down restaurants, remember the acronym S.T.O.P. (**S**low down, **t**ame your appetite, **o**rder wisely, and exercise **p**ortion control.) Once again, the more frequently you dine out, the more you'll need to employ these techniques.

Slow Down

Everyone has experienced that stuffed and uncomfortable feeling that comes from eating too much, too quickly. It doesn't exactly lend itself to a good night's sleep or an overwhelming desire to go out and exercise vigorously, does it? At your next opportunity, try to break this familiar cycle. You've heard these techniques before, but this time, *use* them. One at a time, all at once, whatever works for you—just do it! Put your fork down between bites. Drink water or a nonalcoholic, low-calorie beverage between mouthfuls. Take time to savor every bite and enjoy the conversation at your table. Push your plate aside when you are finished with half and take inventory. Does the food taste as good as it did at the first bite? Do you really want to finish it *now*? Could you take the rest home? Tell yourself, "I can eat this later if I really want to." By the time you get home, you'll feel satisfied with the amount you finished and glad that you can save your leftovers for lunch tomorrow.

Tame Your Appetite

How many times have you "budgeted" your calories for a special evening out only to wait for more than an hour to be seated, another 30 minutes to have your order taken, and in the meantime polished off the entire breadbasket like a ravenous wolf? It's not a good situation for the health-conscious diner, to be sure. Instead of stepping into that trap again, have a small snack before you go out for the evening. An apple with a tablespoon of peanut butter, a cup of yogurt, or a handful of homemade trail mix can be just enough to take the edge off your appetite, but not so much that it spoils your dinner. Remember the Hunger/Fullness Scale introduced in Chapter 3, "Uncover the Natural Eater"? The point is to be eating dinner when you are moderately hungry, not famished.

Order Wisely

Don't be afraid to ask (graciously) for items or combinations not specifically listed on the menu. Ask if low-fat or low-calorie options are available. Ask the server to describe preparation methods. You can almost always substitute steamed vegetables for chips or fries. Order a salad with dressing on the side. Check out Figure 7.1 for more specific recommendations about menu items. Restaurant staffs are usually more than willing to accommodate a courteous, inquisitive customer!

FIGURE 7.1
Familiarize your-
self with menu
lingo.

Beverages

Choose more often:	**Choose less often:**
Water, juice, low-fat milk, coffee, unsweetened iced tea	Whole milk, milkshakes, regular soft drinks, alcohol

Salads

Choose more often:	**Choose less often:**
Toss green salad with vegetable toppings and fat free or vinegar dressing, fresh fruit salad, grilled chicken salad	Potato salad, coleslaw, taco salad shell, regular dressing, olives, cheese, eggs, nuts, croutons, Caesar salad

Bread

Choose more often:	**Choose less often:**
Plain breads, rolls, bread sticks, French bread, bagels	Sweet rolls, muffins, biscuits, croissants, doughnuts

Potatoes and Starches

Choose more often:	**Choose less often:**
Baked, boiled or mashed potatoes, corn, rice, pasta (without cream/butter sauces)	French fries, au gratin, scalloped or hash browned potatoes, potatoes with sauces or gravies

Vegetables

Choose more often:	**Choose less often:**
Boiled, baked, or steamed vegetables	Fried, au gratin, or creamed vegetables, vegetables with sauces or gravies

Entrees

Choose more often:	**Choose less often:**
Baked, roasted or broiled: fish, poultry, lean beef, veal, lamb, pork, pasta with marinara sauce, pizza with vegetable toppings	Fried or breaded meats, casseroles, meats with gravy or sauces, pasta with white or cream sauces, eggs, sausage, bacon, quiche, hash

Portion Control

Most restaurants serve enough food on one plate to last several meals, and most diners clean their plates before giving themselves enough time to feel satisfied or to even enjoy the textures and flavors of the food. In fact, studies show that people actually consume about 56% more food when served extra large portions! In light of this information, you may want to employ some portion control techniques. Order an appetizer and a salad instead of an entree. Ask for half or lunch portions. Start with a cup of broth-based soup—research suggests it may reduce the amount of calories you consume for the total meal. See the following section, "Top Ten Tips for Dining Out the Healthy Way," for more ideas on portion control.

Top Ten Tips for Dining Out the Healthy Way

10. Balance is key. If you know you are going out for a special dinner, have a light lunch (and don't forget a snack before you go). Try getting a little extra physical activity that day.

9. Be familiar with the menu. It can be overwhelming to try to make healthy choices when confronted with an enticing eight-page spread! If you've never been to the restaurant, call ahead to get information about what is offered and how dishes are prepared or check to see whether the establishment offers nutrition information on its website.

8. Order first. You won't be influenced by your companions' choices.

7. Ask your server to remove the bread or tortilla chips from the table after you have taken a small helping. Many people find it difficult to stop eating these types of foods!

6. Split an entree with a friend and order two green side salads. If you're dining alone, ask your server to divide your meal in half and place part of it in a take-home container before it even gets to the table. If you can't take the leftovers with you, ask the server to remove your plate as soon as you are satisfied, or cover the remaining food with a napkin and push the plate away. Remember that it is just as wasteful to consume food that you don't need as it is to throw it away.

5. Avoid regular soft drinks. They're packed with calories and devoid of essential nutrients. Order diet soft drinks if you must, or choose water with lemon, unsweetened iced tea, hot tea, coffee, or low-fat milk instead.

4. Avoid alcohol or limit yourself to one serving—a 4 to 5 ounce glass of wine, 12 ounces of beer, or 1 ounce of hard alcohol. Alcoholic beverages are generally high in calories and can hinder your ability to recognize feelings of fullness.

3. If you are ordering pizza, go for thin crust with lots of vegetables and skip the extra cheese. Add a green salad and you have a complete, balanced meal!

2. Use caution when ordering salads. Though they start well with a base of crisp greens, by the time you add crispy chicken, cheese, bacon, nuts, tortilla strips, croutons, and dressing, you may be looking at more than half your daily calorie needs!

1. Understand serving sizes. The difference between 4 ounces and 8 ounces of prime rib is more than 400 calories. Most people perceive the standard dish of salad dressing as only 2 tablespoons—it's actually four or more—a difference of 150 to 200 calories. As soon as your dinner arrives, divide your plate into at least two portions. That way, you'll have a visual cue to pause midway through the meal to evaluate your body's signals.

To put these techniques in perspective, take a look at the following menu highlights of general categories of restaurants. Dining out frequently can make it difficult to balance your daily calorie intake with your calorie expenditure, so try to choose reasonable meals, and save the "ripoffs" for occasional treats!

Italian Cuisine

Reasonable

> Minestrone soup
>
> Chicken and vegetables
>
> Breadstick (ask for "dry" breadsticks)
>
> Water or tea with lemon

Ripoff

> Fettuccine Alfredo
>
> Breadstick
>
> Salad with regular dressing
>
> 16 oz. soft drink

Tips

The following can be reasonable choices if you save at least one third for later:

- Spaghetti with marinara or meat sauce
- Linguine with marinara or red clam sauce
- Shrimp primavera
- Pasta with tomatoes
- Grilled "catch of the day" with side of vegetables
- Chicken Marsala

Mexican Fare

Reasonable

> Handful of chips with salsa
>
> 2 soft chicken tacos
>
> 1/2 cup refried beans
>
> Water or iced tea

Ripoff

Cheese nachos

Taco salad with sour cream and guacamole (This seemingly healthful selection packs more than 1,000 calories if you eat the shell!)

16 oz. soft drink

Tips

Ask for substitute sides:

- Nonfried pinto or black beans
- Plain salads or steamed veggies
- Salsa, pico de gallo, salsa verde, or hot sauce instead of cheese or sour cream
- Skip the tortilla chips (or have one helping and ask the server to remove the basket)

Succulent Seafood

Reasonable

Blackened catfish

Tossed salad with light dressing

Baked potato with 1 tablespoon sour cream

Water or diet cola

Ripoff

Fried seafood combo with tartar sauce

Tossed salad with regular dressing

Biscuit with butter

French fries

16 oz. soft drink

Tips

Other reasonable choices include

- Broiled or grilled scallops, shrimp, cod, sole, tilapia, trout, flounder, pollock
- Steamed mussels in broth or white wine sauce
- Shrimp scampi—If you leave most of the sauce on the plate!
- Salmon—Save a bit for later

Sides:

- Opt for a dinner roll instead of biscuits.
- Skip the fries and ask for veggies instead.

Guiltless Grills

Reasonable

Grilled chicken

Baked potato with 1 tablespoon sour cream

Vegetable

Iced tea with lemon

Ripoff

Stuffed potato skins with sour cream

Mushroom cheeseburger with onion rings

16 oz. soft drink

Tips

Make a meal of

- A bowl of chili or soup with salad and a roll
- Shrimp cocktail with a salad, veggie, and bread

Other lean choices include

- Sirloin steak
- Grilled/broiled fish

Stake Out the Steak House

Reasonable

Filet mignon (trimmed)

Baked potato with 1 tablespoon sour cream

Vegetable

Water with lemon

Ripoff

> Fried onion with dipping sauce
>
> Prime rib, untrimmed
>
> Caesar salad
>
> Baked potato with butter
>
> 16 oz. soft drink

Tips

Other reasonable picks:

- Barbecued chicken breast
- Sirloin steak
- "Catch of the day"

Sensible sides:

- Baked sweet potato (ask for the toppings on the side)
- Mixed green salad with light dressing
- Veggies (as always)
- Broth-based soup

Asian Alternatives

Reasonable

> Hot & sour soup
>
> Szechuan shrimp
>
> Fortune cookie

Ripoff

> 2 egg rolls
>
> Sweet 'n sour pork
>
> 16 oz. soft drink

Tips

- Try sushi instead.
- Order steamed instead of stir-fried rice.
- Order extra vegetables to mix with your entree, and take some home.
- Beef with broccoli, shrimp with garlic, and chicken chow mein can be decent choices if you save some for later.
- Use chopsticks to slow down and leave some sauce behind.

Morning Meals

Reasonable

Oatmeal with skim, 1%, or 2% milk and fresh fruit

Scrambled egg substitute

Coffee or tea

Ripoff

Pancakes with syrup and margarine

Sausage links

Large orange juice

Tips

- Many establishments offer egg substitutes and "lite" breakfasts (usually toast or bagel, fresh fruit, and scrambled egg substitute).
- Order a la carte or "short stacks" instead of combo platters.
- Canadian bacon, ham, cold cereal, fresh fruit, whole-wheat toast, skim milk, and even soymilk are often available!

Nutrition Tips for Travelers

Traveling for work or pleasure and eating on the go is a way of life for many. Being away from home often disrupts your routine and puts stress on your body, but with a little information and planning, you really can make wiser choices and travel with all your healthy habits:

- Plan ahead. Don't get trapped by limited, unhealthy choices. Travelers often resort to fast food and airport snack bars, sapping their wallets and energy levels for high-fat, low-nutrient foods. Bring along a bag of healthy goodies and snacks to break the cycle. See Figure 7.2 for travel-friendly nutrition.

■ Call the airline ahead of time and request a special meal, such as low sodium or vegetarian. You'll enjoy lighter fare *and* get served first!

■ Bring a small cooler for road trips. Stock it with low-fat yogurt, whole-wheat crackers, fruit, slices of low-fat cheese, baby carrots, cut vegetables, and water.

■ Vacations and conferences often mean constant access to less than perfect meals. Indulge occasionally, but be sure to balance it out with healthy food choices throughout the rest of your day. Your stomach will thank you! Enjoy the fish and chips in London for lunch, and have a broth-based cup of soup and a salad for dinner. Then make the most of pedestrian friendly cities and go for long walks whenever you can.

■ Start your days with a power breakfast to keep your energy up and your hunger level down throughout the morning. Try cereal with skim milk or yogurt, fresh fruit, and chopped almonds; whole-wheat toast with preserves, a hard-cooked egg or scrambled egg substitute, and fruit or juice; or hot oatmeal with walnuts and dried fruit. These morning menus provide complex carbohydrates, moderate amounts of protein, and a little fat to fuel your body for the full day ahead.

■ Avoid the mini bars in hotel rooms. High-calorie alcoholic beverages may help you relax, but they also relax your resolve to eat healthfully away from home. Plunge into your bag of healthy snacks and bottled water; or make your own mixer with club soda and fresh lime juice.

■ Leave your emergency food stash at home? Take a few minutes and go to the nearest grocery store or market to get some healthy supplies for your stay. Whole-grain English muffins, fruit, dried fruit, peanut butter, milk, popcorn, granola bars, precut veggies, and low-fat dip are all good staples while on the road.

■ Eat when you are physically hungry. Many people eat while traveling because they are jet-lagged, dehydrated, tired, frustrated, bored, or lonely. Instead of using food to manage these situations, go for a swim in the hotel's pool or take a stroll through town. Exposure to bright sunlight can help reset your body's internal clock if you're groggy. Bring some good reading material or stationery and catch up on correspondence.

■ Drink plenty of water. Air and road travel can dehydrate you, making you feel tired, sick, cranky, and vulnerable to snack attacks. Aim for eight 8-ounce glasses of water a day, and more if you are traveling in hot climates.

■ Traveling doesn't mean leaving your healthy habits at home! Aim for at least two fruits and three vegetables daily.

FIGURE 7.2

Packing for healthy meals away from home.

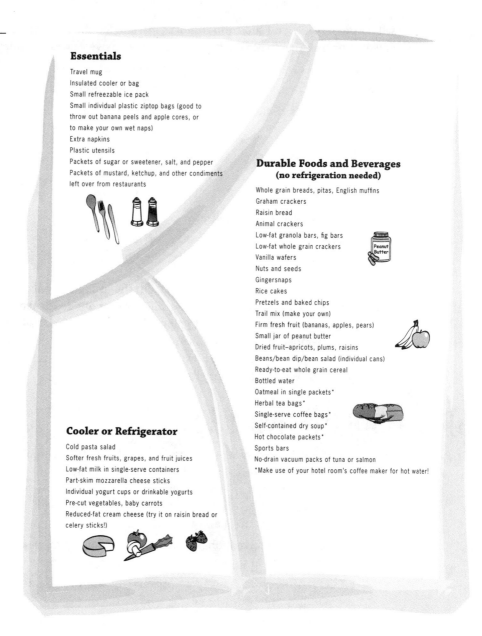

Essentials

Travel mug

Insulated cooler or bag

Small refreezable ice pack

Small individual plastic ziptop bags (good to throw out banana peels and apple cores, or to make your own wet naps)

Extra napkins

Plastic utensils

Packets of sugar or sweetener, salt, and pepper

Packets of mustard, ketchup, and other condiments left over from restaurants

Durable Foods and Beverages
(no refrigeration needed)

Whole grain breads, pitas, English muffins

Graham crackers

Raisin bread

Animal crackers

Low-fat granola bars, fig bars

Low-fat whole grain crackers

Vanilla wafers

Nuts and seeds

Gingersnaps

Rice cakes

Pretzels and baked chips

Trail mix (make your own)

Firm fresh fruit (bananas, apples, pears)

Small jar of peanut butter

Dried fruit–apricots, plums, raisins

Beans/bean dip/bean salad (individual cans)

Ready-to-eat whole grain cereal

Bottled water

Oatmeal in single packets*

Herbal tea bags*

Single-serve coffee bags*

Self-contained dry soup*

Hot chocolate packets*

Sports bars

No-drain vacuum packs of tuna or salmon

*Make use of your hotel room's coffee maker for hot water!

Cooler or Refrigerator

Cold pasta salad

Softer fresh fruits, grapes, and fruit juices

Low-fat milk in single-serve containers

Part-skim mozzarella cheese sticks

Individual yogurt cups or drinkable yogurts

Pre-cut vegetables, baby carrots

Reduced-fat cream cheese (try it on raisin bread or celery sticks!)

A Note on Air Travel

Look into your carrier's food services; some major airlines are discontinuing meal options in economy seating due to time, space, and budget constraints, but many sell gourmet meals and substantial snacks instead. Do the best you can, drink plenty of water, and resolve to eat healthfully when you arrive at your destination!

If alternative meals are offered, you might be able to choose from the following:

▨ Diabetic	▨ Low purine
▨ Low fat, low cholesterol	▨ Gluten-free
▨ Low sodium	▨ Soft diet
▨ Low protein	▨ Peanut-free
▨ High fiber	▨ Children's menu
▨ Asian vegetarian	▨ Low calorie
▨ Lacto-ovo vegetarian or vegan	▨ Kosher
▨ Fruit plates	▨ Sandwiches
▨ Hindu	▨ Muslim

Each airline is different, so be sure to check out the in-flight service section of the airline's website, or call customer service for more information. To take advantage of these special meals, call the airline to place your request at least 24–48 hours in advance. Remember to identify yourself to the gate agent and the flight attendant as you board the plane to let them know you'll be receiving a special meal. Courtesy pays big dividends when it comes to receiving good service!

The Absolute Minimum

When dining out frequently was a luxury enjoyed only by the wealthy few, it wasn't nearly as important for the average diner to be on her "nutritional toes" when choosing meals. In today's culture of convenience, long work weeks, and less leisure time, however, it pays to be a conscientious consumer. When you dine out, travel, or just want to grab a quick meal on the go, remember to

- Seek nutrition information—There's nothing worse than making what you believe to be a healthy choice only to discover the opposite.
- S.T.O.P.—**S**low down; **t**ame your appetite (before you go); **o**rder wisely; and use **p**ortion control strategies!
- Plan ahead—Think about what will be available and make a flexible decision before you get to your destination.
- Be prepared—Bring food with you when you travel, or stop at a grocery store when you arrive. It saves money and time, increases your productivity and energy level, and improves your health.

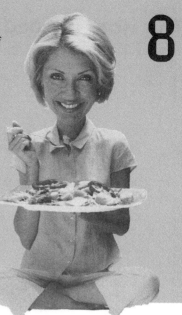

8

HEALTH IS A FAMILY AFFAIR

Family dynamics have an enormous impact on overall health; regardless of the form your family takes, interactions within the context of this unit influence your daily eating and activity patterns. This chapter is devoted to helping you understand your role in creating an environment that supports healthy eating and activity choices for every family member. Even if you live alone, these concepts can be applied to your responsibility to care for *yourself* in a thoughtful manner.

Your Role in Feeding a Family

Do any of these statements sound familiar?

"You can eat your cookies after you've finished your broccoli."

"You're not leaving the table until you clean your plate, and that's final."

"But Da-ad, I *hate* green beans!"

"Honey, if you just behave a little longer, you can have ice cream when we get home."

Ready to reach for the pain reliever yet? These statements represent common interactions when it comes to parents, children, and food. Unfortunately, the current culture dictates negative attitudes when it comes to providing food for yourself and your loved ones. Take a look at some of the most common problematic family feeding patterns:

- Some parents seemingly do a decent job of feeding their children but fail to treat themselves with the same care. They get a meal on the table as soon as possible after work but don't even sit down with their children to eat it! They might stand at the counter, pay bills, or talk on the phone, but their children are left to fend for themselves. Late at night, after bedtime, the exhausted parents finally stop to eat something themselves—snack foods, ice cream, chips—whatever they can find that requires little preparation. Children in these families don't have the reinforcement and support they need (through a positive eating role model) to become independent with their food intake and frequently become "picky eaters." They eat a limited variety of familiar foods and demand that their parents essentially become short-order cooks, preparing macaroni and cheese for one child, chicken nuggets for another, and peanut butter and jelly for the third.

- Many families are involved in so many activities that the family meal seems like an ancient relic from a time long before cell phones, the Internet, pagers, and voice mail made people accessible 24 hours a day. Parents in these families might *want* to live differently but just never seem to be able to disengage from the endless stream of activities and responsibilities that characterize life in the twenty-first century. Health and well-being (of parents *and* children) suffer as meals take a back burner to practices, meetings, games, performances, and other events. The problem isn't necessarily the activities themselves but the way in which they displace the family meal and simply spending time together.

■ Many parents have uncomfortable relationships with food and eating them-selves—they believe they know what they "should" be eating, but because this seldom happens, they feel guilty and anxious about food, meals, and snacks. They might be frequent dieters, constantly losing and gaining the same 10, 20, or 30 pounds (or more) and speaking negatively about their own bodies. Or they might be concerned about a pudgy child and, although genuinely trying to do what's best for him or her, become overly restrictive in providing food for the child. Children in these families often develop a keen interest in "junk food" because it becomes their forbidden fruit. Food battles revolve around what they can and can't have, and what children are eating when parents aren't around to police their food choices.

Unfortunately, the three previous scenarios are the rule instead of the exception, and they often produce children, teens, and adults who aren't fully capable of regulating their food intake in a relaxed, healthful, and moderate fashion. You have probably been doing your level best to provide good food for your family, but if you honestly evaluate the eating environment in your home, you might find that something (or everything!) is missing. There is a better way, but it takes some thought, flexible dis-cipline, and a willingness to experiment with new behaviors and attitudes. If you are responsible for providing food for and raising children, you have a unique opportunity to nurture their ability to regulate food intake internally so that food assumes its appropriate place in their lives. What an awesome responsibility!

To achieve this lofty goal without putting too much pressure on yourself or your loved ones, you must understand that each player has certain responsibilities. These change and grow as your family grows, but it is critical that you fully accept the uniqueness of your respective roles. This *division of responsibility* with regard to feed-ing (see Figure 8.1), the brainchild of Ellyn Satter, MS, RD, LCSW, BCD, can make a world of difference in your family's eating experiences. This chapter can put you on the right track, but if you and/or your children are struggling with food and eating issues, Satter's three books—*Child of Mine, Feeding with Love and Good Sense*; *How to Get Your Kid to Eat...But Not Too Much*; and *Secrets of Feeding a Healthy Family*—and her website www.ellynsatter.com are invaluable resources. Don't delay seeking pro-fessional assistance if you feel it's warranted. These issues have an enormous impact on your overall health and well being, and that of your children.

FIGURE 8.1

The division of
responsibility in
early childhood.
Reprinted with
permission from
Ellyn Satter's
*Secrets of Feeding
a Healthy Family*
(Kelcy Press,
1999).

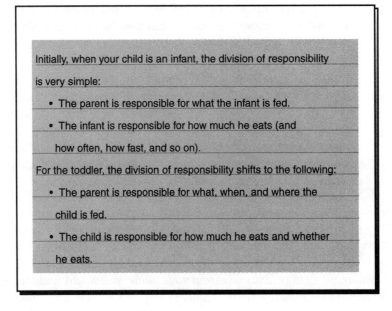

Initially, when your child is an infant, the division of responsibility
is very simple:

- The parent is responsible for what the infant is fed.
- The infant is responsible for how much he eats (and
  how often, how fast, and so on).

For the toddler, the division of responsibility shifts to the following:

- The parent is responsible for what, when, and where the
  child is fed.
- The child is responsible for how much he eats and whether
  he eats.

As your child moves beyond the toddler years, the division of responsibility continues to transform, but it's critical that you realize the value of supporting your older children by continuing to provide wholesome meals at predictable times and to *be there* to eat them together as a family. In *Secrets of Feeding a Healthy Family*, Satter says

> As your child gets older, he will become more independent. He may seem so independent, in fact, that you may forget how important you as parent continue to be. An 11- or 13-year-old child can make his own sandwich or even warm up his own food. In many families, older children get home first and even eat before parents arrive. Food companies capitalize on this trend with 'meals for children' or 'cooking classes for kids.' They want to convince you that feeding is a do-it-yourself business so you'll buy their products. It's not. Your children still need you to feed them.

You might be thinking, "what kind of crazy plan is *that*?" You might be relieved to learn that you don't have to control your child's eating; you might feel apprehensive about letting go of that control; or you might be dreading fulfilling some of your responsibilities. All these responses are perfectly normal and valid. Feeding your family is a trial-and-error kind of process, and you can expect to make many mistakes along the way. The important thing is that you are willing to observe the state of your family's current food environment and make adjustments if they are warranted.

Satter goes on to describe some of the parents' tasks with regard to feeding:

> For children to do a good job with eating, parents and other adults have to do certain things to support them. Those tasks include providing food, making eating times pleasant and predictable, and showing your child what it means to grow up with regard to eating.

When you fully accept these tasks and allow your children to perform *their own* eating jobs, mealtime becomes a pleasure instead of a nuisance, a headache, or an all-out power struggle.

Provide Good Food

Providing meals for your family is actually far less complicated than it seems. You don't need to be a gourmet cook or spend hours planning menus and shopping for ingredients to prepare elaborate recipes. Good meals are different for every family, but at a minimum, they should be safe to eat (see Chapter 9, "In the Kitchen 101"), include tasty foods, and contain a variety of foods from each of the five main food groups (see Chapter 5, "Putting It Together—Real Food for Real People"). This leaves plenty of wiggle room for fast foods, convenience foods, and eating at restaurants occasionally. Take a look at the following list for examples of quick, reasonably nutritious meals that use some prepared foods:

- Boxed macaroni and cheese with frozen broccoli and carrot coins thrown in with the pasta during the last few minutes of cooking. Serve with drained canned peaches and milk.

- Frozen vegetable lasagna, cooked, served with bagged tossed salad and dressing, grapes, and milk.

- Fast food hamburgers served with cut up vegetables and fruit from the deli (carrots, broccoli, pepper strips, sliced apples, pineapple, and so on). These go over well when paired with favorite dips—peanut butter, yogurt, salad dressing, honey mustard—whatever your family enjoys!

- Angel hair pasta (cooks in 4 minutes flat) with jarred chunky marinara sauce, Parmesan cheese, and/or drained canned chicken, tuna, or salmon. Serve with a green salad mixed with orange or apple sections and topped with dressing.

■ For a light meal, serve toasted frozen waffles with a buffet of toppings—flavored yogurt, cut-up fruit, peanut butter, syrup, low-fat granola, and so on. Round it out with milk and juice to drink.

Many people become so paralyzed by nutrition messages in the media that they quit trying altogether. They feel so guilty about their food choices that they take the all-or-nothing approach—they're either being "good" (preparing labor-intensive, ultra-nutritious meals), or they're being "bad" (stopping by fast food restaurants for the whole nine yards five days a week). Sometimes, the best thing to do is relax your standards, use a few favorite convenience foods, and try your best to fill in the nutritional gaps. Chapter 9 goes into more detail about food preparation and cooking techniques, *if* you are interested.

Make Eating Times Pleasant and Predictable

The current health culture places so much emphasis on *what* to eat (or avoid) that most people have forgotten *how* to eat. Mealtime often occurs in the family car between practices and games, after 8 o'clock at night, or not at all. Children and parents eat in shifts, with each family member fending for him- or herself whenever the opportunity arises. Adults never sit down to eat a real meal; they graze their way through the day, snatching food from vending machines, candy jars on co-workers' desks, or leftovers from a child's plate. These same adults raise children who have never truly seen or experienced relaxed, healthy, normal eating.

If you're reading this chapter thinking, "I know this is important, but there just isn't time," or "sitting down to a family meal four or five times a week is completely unrealistic," I strongly encourage you to consider the costs you and your children are paying when you don't make family meals a priority. A recent study (*Archives of Pediatric and Adolescent Medicine, 2004*) concluded that children who eat regular meals with their parents are less likely to

■ Use tobacco, alcohol, and marijuana

■ Have low grade point averages

■ Display symptoms of depression

■ Have suicidal involvement

What is keeping you from eating meals together as a family (or sitting down to a meal yourself)? Is it over-involvement in after-school activities, sports, or clubs? Do you spend too much time and energy at work? Are volunteer commitments taking over your evenings? As noble as many of these activities are, *none of them* can replace simply sitting down with your family and sharing a meal. The content of that meal is less important than the commitment to making it happen. Be as consistent as possible. Aim for having dinner around the same time each evening so that all parties involved know what to expect. You can plan an afternoon snack that helps keep the peace, so to speak, but establishing a consistent mealtime goes a long way toward nurturing healthy eating habits for parents and children alike.

To make mealtime as pleasant as possible, respect the division of responsibility. You are responsible for getting the meal on the table (children can help, within reason), and each person that sits down is responsible for deciding whether, what, and how much to eat of what you have provided. Got that? No short-order cooking; no separate meals for picky eaters. It helps to have some familiar food on the table at every meal—perhaps bread or crackers with a selection of spreads, fruit, salad, or whatever works for your family—so that even picky eaters can fall back on something. Research and experience have shown that children need to be exposed to a new food *at least* nine or ten times before they will successfully chew and swallow it. It is your responsibility to do the exposing (and be a good role model), and the child's responsibility to learn to eat.

Finally, do what you can to provide a pleasant atmosphere. That means many different things to many different families. For some, it might include lighting candles and using real napkins. For others, the thought of doing all those dishes and laundry spoils the entire eating experience. Use Figure 8.2 to spark your imagination when it comes to enjoying family mealtime.

note

If you are interested in changing your family's eating habits, be prepared for resistance. The older your children, the more difficult these changes will be. You might want to hold a family conference to let them know what you are planning on doing and why to give them an opportunity to ask questions and clarify what will be expected of them. Younger children will adapt more quickly but might still benefit from being told about the coming changes. You are the parent, and you decide which changes make the most sense in your unique family.

FIGURE 8.2

Make meals more enjoyable!

Light candles

Use real napkins and silverware

Use paper plates and plastic silverware to minimize clean–up time

Play soothing music

Turn off the TV

Let each person at the table relay a story from his/her day

Take a moment to be thankful for the food you're about to eat and a

    home in which to eat it

Don't discuss worrisome topics at the table

Don't force your child to eat anything

Teach children how to decline food politely (no "Ewww,

    broccoli!" or "That's disgusting!")

Delegate mealtime tasks to each family member

Pause halfway through the meal to assess how you're feeling internally

Dim the lights

Eat outside

Clear the table of miscellaneous papers, bills, etc.

Take your time

Plan dessert into the meal instead of relegating it to late-night

    "forbidden food"

Be a Good Role Model

Your children must not only be told what is expected of them with regard to appropriate eating habits, they must see you do it! This is the best way for children to "grow up" with food. If they see mom and dad skipping meals, they will, too. If you have ice cream every night, it's a sure bet they will expect the same. If you offer sweets as a reward, they will learn that food makes difficult tasks more tolerable.

Children have a way of galvanizing every belief you hold dear; they become the mirror in which you see yourself more clearly. If you truly believe that healthy, moderate eating is important, work on your own eating habits first. Parents who are relaxed and confident with food raise children who are interested in eating, who know how to try new foods or decline them politely, and who respect their own tastes and bodies.

Become an Active Family!

So far in this chapter, you've learned about the dynamics of feeding your children, but this discussion would be incomplete without addressing the need for more physically active families. Unfortunately, just as sit-down meals have become the exception, so has the number of families who incorporate an appropriate amount of regular physical activity. We're not talking about bringing your kids to the gym and pumping iron together, either. This is simply moving more and sitting less, and encouraging your loved ones to do the same.

Reduce Sedentary Time

As with nutrition, many parents become so overwhelmed with recommendations about exercise that they do nothing. They feel like they won't get any good out of doing less than 60 minutes of heart-pounding activity five days a week, so they avoid the issue altogether and choose to relax by watching TV, surfing the Internet, going out to eat, renting movies, or catching up on email. There's nothing wrong with any one of these activities, per se, but when they compose the majority of your family's leisure time, everyone's health and well-being suffers.

Chart your sedentary behaviors for a week (see Figure 8.3) to see how quickly they add up. Ask your kids to do the same. When you realize you (or your children) are watching an average of two to three hours of television a day, it becomes clear that you *do have* the time to be active together. Set time limits on some of your family's major sedentary behaviors and keep track of them in a public place on a dry erase board. When an individual reaches the limit, it's time to go outside, read, play games, or go for a walk or bike ride.

By limiting these types of activities, you'll begin to open the door to a more active lifestyle. Don't expect to be popular for instituting this kind of change, but stick with it and watch as the entire family reaps the benefits.

FIGURE 8.3

How many minutes per day/week do you spend in each of the following activities?

Talking on the phone

Sitting at a desk

Working on a computer

Playing computer or video games

Watching television

Watching movies

Emailing or instant messaging

Surfing the Web

Driving/commuting

Sitting in class

Limit Extracurricular Involvement

Another major barrier to being active together as a family is the abundance of groups, clubs, teams, and lessons available to people of all ages. Being involved in meaningful activities is important, but being overwhelmed by conflicting schedules, limited resources (and limited drivers, for that matter), and overbooked calendars benefits no one. Realistically assess the activities in which you and your children participate—sit down first with your partner and then as a family to discuss which are most important and which have become burdensome. No one else can do this for you, and no one can tell you the "right" level of involvement for your particular situation. Just remember that the best intentions to become more active are meaningless if there simply isn't enough time to make them happen.

Get Moving!

After you pinpoint and reduce sedentary behaviors and streamline your family's extracurricular involvement, it's time to get moving. If you don't know where to begin, start with an after-dinner walk. In Italy, evening strolls are simply part of the culture. During the *passegiata* (literally "wandering"), men, women, and children of all ages stroll leisurely through town and city streets, meeting and greeting each other as they go. You don't have to be Italian or live in a beautiful Tuscan hill town to enjoy this wonderful custom. Make it part of your own family's culture, and your children will come to enjoy it and the time that you spend together.

Other families prefer more competitive activities. Head outside after dinner to shoot baskets, play football, or throw a Frisbee. If you don't have enough space in the yard, save the competitive games for the weekends and then head for the nearest public park. One potential challenge with these types of activities is that different children have different levels of athletic ability. If you have a "nonathlete" in your family, it's critical to do things together that don't require great athletic prowess. Long bike rides, hiking, playing on a playground, and dancing are inclusive activities that can help less physically fit or sport-oriented children (and parents) feel comfortable with and confident in their bodies.

Weekends and vacations offer a unique opportunity to plan physical activity into your family's schedule. One of my favorite memories from childhood is that of the family camping trip. Once a year or so, we loaded our pop-up camper, hitched it to the family wagon or van, and headed to a state park for a few days. We hiked, swam, or sledded, depending on the season; fixed our meals on the campfire; and just generally had a ball. I'm sure there were many trips that went smoothly, but it's the disastrous ones that emblazon themselves in the memory and make for fun stories when you get older. If you've never tried it before, borrow someone's tent and give it a shot—what do you have to lose? Check out Figure 8.4 for more ideas on getting your family moving.

Play Twister

Have a hula hoop contest

Play hopscotch

Jump rope

Fly a kite

Draw a course on your driveway with sidewalk chalk

Walk around the block

Pack a picnic, and don't forget the football or Frisbee

Ride your bikes to the nearest basketball court or playground

Let each child have a small garden—plant tomatoes,

    herbs, peppers, beans, flowers, etc.

Rake leaves together and jump in them

In winter, go ice skating, sledding, cross-country skiing, or make

    a snowman/fort

Frequent "you pick" farms for strawberries, blueberries, apples, etc.

Play hide and seek

Go inline skating on sidewalks or greenways (remember the

    safety gear!)

Wash the dog

Wash the car

Go bowling

THE ABSOLUTE MINIMUM

- Become aware of your family's current feeding patterns.
- Accept responsibility for your tasks as parent—you determine the when, where, and what of eating.
- Allow your children to do their jobs—they determine whether and how much to eat.
- Make mealtimes as pleasant as possible by observing the division of responsibility and by providing meals consistently—experiment with ways to make the eating atmosphere enjoyable.
- Become aware of and set limits on sedentary behaviors in your home—for all members of the family.
- Evaluate your level of involvement in extracurricular activities and make changes if necessary.
- Seek physical activities that include each family member.
- Plan active weekends and vacations.

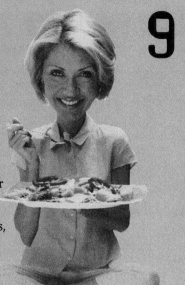

9

- Food safety basics—if it isn't safe to eat, the nutrition content doesn't matter

- Be prepared—a bit about meal planning and stocking your kitchen with the essential tools and equipment

- Know your kitchen vocabulary—a primer on the most common cooking techniques

- Season foods well with herbs, spices, and other tasty additions

- Recipe modification—lighten up your favorites, or decide to leave well enough alone

IN THE KITCHEN 101

"Cooking" can have a positive or a negative connotation, depending on your upbringing, culture, personal experiences, dieting history, and many other factors. Plenty of you probably feel confident in your culinary skills but are looking for new ways to cook and modify recipes that reflect a healthier lifestyle. For some of you, the task of food preparation seems like an incredible bore—"cooking" is a nuisance you'd just as soon pass along to someone else. And there are likely many of you who take the middle road—you wouldn't mind cooking if you had a little extra time and some basic skills. Regardless of your past kitchen experience, this chapter is designed to ensure that you understand some fundamental concepts about food preparation, cooking techniques, and recipe modification.

Keep Food Safe

Ah, yes, the scintillating topic of food safety. It's something you don't think about much until you've eaten food that *isn't* safe and pay the consequences for a day or two. Although food safety doesn't exactly knock your socks off, it is definitely one of the most important skills you can practice. If you are responsible for preparing food for children, elderly relatives or friends, or people with compromised immune systems, this issue can be as serious as life or death. By following a few simple rules (and yes, these are rules, not guidelines), you can ensure that the food you eat and provide is as safe as possible.

Avoid the Danger Zone

The *Danger Zone* refers to a temperature range—specifically 40° to 140° Fahrenheit—that provides the ideal environment for rapid growth of harmful bacteria, the primary culprits in food-borne illnesses.

To keep food out of the Danger Zone, observe the following:

- Ensure that hot food stays hot (think steamy hot and bubbling around the edges) and cold food stays cold (below 40°).
- Never leave food sitting out at room temperature for more than two hours total, including preparation, transport, and serving time.
- Ensure that you cook foods to the proper temperatures to destroy harmful bacteria (see Table 9.1).
- Cool cooked food quickly by refrigerating it first in a shallow dish and then transferring to storage containers if necessary.
- Thaw most frozen foods in the refrigerator, not on the kitchen counter, and keep raw meats, poultry, and seafood on the bottom shelf in a separate pan to prevent juices from dripping and contaminating other food items. Some foods can be thawed with cold running water, and if so, the packaging should state more specific directions.
- Keep calibrated thermometers in your refrigerator and freezer to ensure proper storage temperatures. Keep your refrigerator between 34° and 40° F. If you plan to store foods for long periods of time (more than a few months) in a freezer, keep it at 0° or colder. If you can't get your freezer temperature that low, plan to cycle through foods stored there more quickly.

TABLE 9.1 Proper Cooking Temperatures

Product	°F
Eggs & Egg Dishes	
Eggs	Cook until yolk and white are firm
Egg dishes	160
Ground Meat & Meat Mixtures	
Turkey, chicken	165
Veal, beef, lamb, pork	160
Beef	
Medium rare	145
Medium	160
Well done	170
Veal	
Medium rare	145
Medium	160
Well done	170
Lamb	
Medium rare	145
Medium	160
Well done	170
Pork	
Medium	160
Well done	170
Poultry	
Chicken, whole	180
Turkey, whole	180
Poultry breasts, roast	170
Poultry thighs, wings	180
Stuffing (cooked alone or in bird)	165
Duck & goose	180
Ham	
Fresh (raw)	160
Precooked (to reheat)	140

Table 9.1   (Continued)

Product	°F
Seafood	
Fin fish	Cook until opaque and flakes easily with a fork
Shrimp, lobster, crab	Should turn red and flesh should become pearly opaque
Scallops	Should turn milky white or opaque and firm
Clams, mussels, oysters	Cook until shells open

Source: USDA's Food Safety Facts (http://vm.cfsan.fda.gov/~fsg/fs-cook.html)

If you pack perishable food for lunch or snacks, it's best to keep it in an insulated cooler with an ice pack of some sort. Ideally, place the cooler in a refrigerator when you arrive at your destination if it will be more than an hour or two before you eat. Otherwise, feel free to freeze portions of your lunch to keep the rest of the food items cold. Try freezing 100% juice boxes, plastic yogurt pouches, bread for sandwiches, or fruit salad—this may change the texture slightly but helps ensure your food stays safe.

Improper handling of leftovers is a major culprit in many cases of food-borne illness. Keep these tips in mind to avoid becoming a victim in your own kitchen:

- Use leftovers as soon as possible—preferably within one to three days.
- Store them in microwave-safe plastic or glass containers with tightly fitting lids.
- Reheat leftovers *one time only*.
- Arrange foods so that the thickest pieces are toward the edge of the plate or dish and thinner, smaller pieces are in the center.
- When reheating, cover the container with a microwave-safe lid, wax paper, or a paper plate or towel; be sure to vent a corner if using a lid.
- Stir halfway through reheating and check to be sure that leftovers are very hot throughout when finished.

Keep a Clean Kitchen

Simply washing your hands and food preparation surfaces and utensils thoroughly can prevent most food-borne illnesses. Use good technique when washing your hands—use hot water and a mild soap, and work up a good lather, taking care to clean between fingers and underneath your fingernails; rinse well and dry with a clean towel or disposable paper towel. Wash your hands frequently—before preparing food, after handling raw protein-rich foods, after sneezing or wiping your kid's nose, and again before you eat. Keep a sinkful of hot, soapy water available as you cook to wash contaminated utensils and dishes immediately after use. For items that have been in contact with raw poultry, eggs, meat, or seafood, a brief rinse in a chlorine bleach-water solution (approximately 2 teaspoons per quart of water) after washing with soapy water can ensure more complete disinfection. Wet towels, rags, and sponges often become breeding grounds for bacteria, so change them frequently and/or sanitize them in the bleach solution mentioned previously. If you're a bleach fanatic, you might want to purchase white towels and dish rags to avoid unsightly spots on colored linens.

> **tip**
>
> When using a bleach solution to sanitize cooking utensils, wear an apron or old t-shirt to avoid ugly white spots on your favorite clothes, and let the utensils air dry. Don't forget to wear rubber gloves, or you'll get "bleach hands."

Avoid cross contamination by keeping one cutting board and knife for fresh produce and another set for uncooked meats, poultry, and seafood. Another common kitchen mistake is using the same utensils for raw and cooked foods (for example, placing grilled chicken back on the plate used for marinating raw chicken or using the same tongs to transfer raw meat to the pan and cooked meat from the pan to the serving dish). The safest bet is to treat anything that has touched a "dangerous" food item, typically uncooked protein-based foods, as contaminated and put it immediately in the hot, soapy water you prepared ahead of time.

Rinse all fresh produce thoroughly with cold running water—including melon, kiwi, and anything else with a rind or skin you intend to slice. Bacteria from the outside can easily be transferred to the edible portion when cutting these types of fruits. And don't dry produce on a used dish or hand towel—unless you want to introduce new bacteria into your fruit salad.

All right, you've probably had enough, though we've only covered the bare minimum when it comes to food safety. If you follow these rules (remember, these are the only rules in the book—the rest are suggestions and guidelines!), you can eat and provide tasty meals that keep you and your family in good health.

Be a Boy Scout

Anyone interested in eating well and helping his or her family do the same needs to do some planning and be prepared. As tedious as it sounds, planning a week's worth of meals is one of the best ways to get in the routine of healthy cooking and to make sure that you don't get halfway through dinner preparation only to discover you're missing a key ingredient. Meal planning also helps to minimize the familiar "Oh my gosh, it's 7:30! We have nothing to eat in the house; someone better go get carry-out!" syndrome.

If you've never dabbled in meal planning, take a look at the week's supermarket bargains to give you some direction. If planning six or seven meals sounds daunting, start with one or two you'd like to try, and then fill in the gaps with "no recipe needed" nights. These could include simple suppers such as toasted sandwiches and prepared soups, large chef salads with bread and fruit, or homemade "pita pizzas"—the previous chapters are chock-full of no-fuss meal ideas, so reread them if you need some help.

So much information about planning meals and menus is available that I won't go into much depth here, except to encourage you to experiment with meal planning just like you might experiment with new foods. With food, you try a little bit at a time to figure out what you like, and pretty soon, you've developed a mature palate that enjoys hummus and toasted pita wedges, as well as crunchy potato chips. When experimenting with meal planning, start small—perhaps as small as trying one new recipe a month, or committing to preparing a large batch of soup on the weekend to last a few days. With practice, meal planning will become an enjoyable part of your new healthy lifestyle and will make you more efficient in the kitchen.

Many individuals and families find it easier to manage meal planning if they develop some kind of logical pattern that works for their schedules. They might prepare a roast or chicken for Sunday supper and then eat leftovers Monday night. Tuesdays are soup and sandwich nights; if they have a little extra time on Wednesdays, they might tackle a new recipe. Thursdays can be leftovers or based on a prepared frozen entrée, and Fridays are pizza nights. Saturdays can be used for shopping and for doing some advance food preparation. This is a perfect time for preparing fresh vegetables for the week, washing and spinning dry salad greens, making a big bowl of fruit salad, and chopping onions and peppers.

On a much smaller scale, make sure that you prepare yourself and your kitchen well when doing the actual cooking. Read through any recipes you'll be using in their entirety and get out all the necessary ingredients and cooking utensils *before* you begin. Some people even like to do this part the night before or in the morning before they leave for work.

Speaking of ingredients and utensils, have you taken inventory of your kitchen cabinets and drawers lately? Starting with a clean slate can bring some clarity to your cooking and eating habits in unexpected ways. How many wooden spoons or sets of measuring cups have you collected? Do bulky, seldom-used appliances take up all of your storage or counter space? The question to ask is not "will I ever use this?" but "will I use this often enough to justify keeping it?" So go ahead and do it; devote a Saturday afternoon to going through every gadget, appliance, utensil, and dish you can find; get rid of duplicates and unnecessary pieces; and reorganize what's left. Check out the following lists for the essentials. You are welcome to keep an unlisted gadget if you use it at least once a year and if you have the storage space. If an item doesn't meet these two criteria, get ruthless. Ask someone else to get rid of the unused items if you must, but be sure it gets done!

Pots and pans:

- Saucepans with lids (several sizes; one should hold 3 quarts)
- Sauté pan with lid (about same diameter as a large skillet, but deeper)
- Skillets (8 inch and 10 inch, nonstick is practical)
- Stockpot with lid (an 8 quart is pretty versatile)
- Broiler pan (comes with oven)
- Roasting pan (deep and heavy duty)

Knives (if you're going to splurge, do it on these!):

- Paring knife (for small jobs)
- Chef's knife (for almost anything)
- Serrated knife (for tomatoes and hearty breads)
- Sharpening tool

Utensils:

- Measuring spoons
- Dry measuring cups
- Liquid measuring cup (glass is best)
- Two cutting boards (one for produce; one for meats, poultry, and fish)
- Serving spoons (slotted and regular)
- Ladle
- Wooden spoons (two is plenty)
- Rubber spatulas (one or two)
- Pancake turner (hard rubber if you use nonstick pans)
- Tongs
- Grater

- Colander
- Vegetable peeler
- Potato masher
- Can opener
- Wire whisk
- Baster
- Corkscrew
- Salad spinner (maybe not essential, but very handy!)
- Meat mallet
- Zester
- Thermometers (go nuts! one for food, oven, refrigerator, freezer)
- Timer (if your oven doesn't have one)

Bowls, dishes, and storage containers:

- Mixing bowls (three should do it)
- Rectangular glass baking dishes (at least a 9×13 inch and an 8×8 inch)
- Microwave- and oven-safe casseroles with lids
- Airtight containers for leftovers and dry ingredients (flour, sugar, and such)

Miscellaneous baking equipment (not essential for survival, but everyone loves homemade goodies once in a while!):

- One or two round cake pans
- One or two loaf pans
- Baking sheets
- Muffin tin
- Rolling pin
- Cooling racks

Appliances:

- Blender
- Toaster oven or toaster
- Hand or standing mixer
- Slow cooker

Know Your Terms—Cooking Vocabulary

It's amazing how few people understand basic cooking techniques. See the following lists for brief descriptions of some of the most common techniques.

Moist heat methods:

- Boiling—Cooking food, covered or uncovered, in liquid that is bubbling and breaking the surface; commonly used for pasta, starches, and vegetables.

- Braising—Usually begins with browning food in a hot pan, adding a small amount of liquid, covering tightly, and simmering until done; often used for poultry and meats.

- Poaching—Cooking food gently in simmering liquid, usually on the stove top; ideal for eggs and mild fish.

- Stewing—Similar to braising, but with enough liquid to cover the food; commonly used for tougher cuts of meat.

- Steaming—Cooking foods over, not in, about an inch of simmering or boiling water; makes excellent crisp-tender vegetables.

Dry heat methods:

- Baking—Cooking food in a pan or dish using the oven's dry heat; used for breads, muffins, cakes, as well as meat, poultry, and seafood.

- Broiling—Cooking with direct heat; usually refers to heating from above (as in the top element of the oven); thin pieces of meat, seafood, or poultry are delicious broiled.

- Deep frying—Usually involves coating foods with batter or dredging in seasoned flour and cooking by completely immersing in hot fat; nearly any food can be deep fried, but particularly tasty with poultry and seafood.

- Grilling—Cooking with direct heat; usually refers to heating from below (as in the backyard charcoal or gas grill); try basting skewers of vegetables with Italian dressing and grilling alongside your chicken.

- Roasting—Similar to baking, usually with slightly higher temperatures; often used for large cuts of meat or poultry.

- Stir frying—Cooking small, uniform pieces of food in a pan or wok in a bit of oil over very high heat, stirring constantly; properly stir-fried vegetables retain their color and crisp texture beautifully.

If you can master a few basic cooking techniques, you won't need too many recipes, especially if you start with high-quality ingredients. A plain piece of fish can be transformed into a wonderful main dish with a drizzling of olive oil, lemon juice, salt, and chopped fresh basil. Use recipes to get started, but feel free to experiment in the kitchen till your heart and stomach are content!

Flavor Your Foods Well

Herbs and spices add interesting flavors to foods and help reduce the need for excessive amounts of added fat, salt, and sugar. In many recipes that call for sugar, for example, you can reduce the amount by a fourth (or more) and add "sweet spices" such as cinnamon, ginger, nutmeg, and allspice to enhance the sweetness. Don't get carried away with this advice, though. Many people ruin perfectly good recipes by trying to cut out all the fat, salt, and sugar, and end up with unsatisfying results and unhappy diners. These ingredients make foods taste good, and in some cases, are essential to the success of the recipe. Make modifications where it makes sense to you, and use dried and fresh herbs to enhance your recipes instead of to eliminate "unhealthy" ingredients. Use the following list for help in pairing common foods with appropriate seasonings:

- Dips—Oregano, parsley, chives, black pepper, onion or garlic powder, dill
- Salads—Basil, oregano, onion, parsley, sesame seeds, flavored vinegars, lemon, mint, fresh fruit
- Vegetables—Chives, dill, onion, garlic, vinegar, pepper, paprika, marjoram
- Fruits—Cinnamon, mint, cloves, nutmeg, ginger, lemon, onion (think pineapple and peach salsas)
- Beef—Allspice, bay leaf, cayenne pepper, curry powder, garlic, black pepper, mushrooms, onion, sage, red wine
- Pork—Apples, applesauce, cinnamon, cloves, garlic, onion, sage, rosemary, zest or juice of citrus fruits
- Poultry—Basil, garlic, pepper, lemon juice, onion, paprika, lemon pepper, rosemary, sage, thyme, tarragon, white wine, oregano
- Fish and seafood—Allspice, basil, curry powder, garlic, lemon juice, Dijon mustard, green onion, paprika, sage, tarragon, thyme, pepper, dry mustard powder, onion powder, dill
- Soups and stews—Basil, bay leaf, pepper, chili powder, garlic, onion, parsley, peppercorns, vinegar, tarragon, rosemary
- Beans and legumes—Cumin, cayenne pepper, curry powder, onion, garlic, chili powder, pepper, honey, brown sugar

Here are a few simple ideas for using herbs, spices, and various other seasonings in your kitchen:

- Make your own flavored butter. Bring stick butter to room temperature and blend 1/4 cup with
    - A few tablespoons of your favorite fresh herbs; use on cooked vegetables, pasta, and lean fish (store covered in refrigerator).
    - Honey and orange zest (use a fine grater to remove the outermost portion of the orange peel) to taste; use on toast, bagels, muffins, and waffles (store covered in refrigerator).
- Mix sour cream or plain yogurt with peeled, seeded, chopped cucumbers and dill for a dressing for fish or baked potatoes.
- Peel, seed, and chop a small cucumber and place in bowl; with a mortar and pestle, make a paste with a little olive oil, sea salt, minced garlic, and lemon juice. Mix the paste with a cup (more or less as desired) of plain yogurt and combine with the cucumber. Serve with pita bread, fish, potatoes, beef, and lamb.
- Make your own dressing for salad. In a glass jar with a tight-fitting lid, mix olive oil with your favorite vinegar (balsamic is especially good) in a 2 to 1 ratio; add salt and pepper to taste. Variations: Add minced garlic, Dijon mustard, or sugar. Start with just a couple tablespoons of this dressing for a whole bowl of salad and use your scrupulously clean hands to toss it well. Add more dressing or salt if needed.
- Mix a little honey and minced fresh ginger (the jarred variety is easy to use!) with mustard and use as a dip for chicken nuggets or fresh vegetables.
- Stir crushed, drained pineapple into jarred salsa and use as a topping for chicken or fish.
- Make homemade yogurt cheese. This method creates a product that can be used as a tasty base for dips and for topping baked potatoes and chili. Use any plain or flavored yogurt that does not contain gelatin. Line a colander with a coffee filter or double layer of paper towels and set over large bowl or pan; then spoon yogurt into the lined colander. Cover loosely and refrigerate for 8 to 24 hours to let fluid drain. The longer the yogurt drains, the thicker the consistency of the final product. Yogurt drained 8 to 12 hours can be used as a sour cream substitute; yogurt drained for 24 hours can be used in place of cream cheese. Discard the fluid that drains off (or use in soups and stews) and use a spatula to scrape the yogurt cheese into a resealable container. Use flavored yogurts such as vanilla, lemon, or strawberry to make tasty spreads for English muffins, toast, bagels, and waffles.

Modifying Recipes

The problem is rarely a shortage of recipes—many of you probably have at least 10 cookbooks at home gathering dust on a shelf and a pile of recipes you've clipped from newspapers and magazines or printed from the Internet, just waiting to be brought to life. If you've been hoarding recipes for the better part of your adult life, a little spring cleaning may be in order. Ask yourself which cookbooks and recipes you are most likely to actually *use*, and give away the rest. Yes, you might decide to attempt homemade Italian gnocchi someday, but if you do, you can always rely on Internet instructions. If you really don't have a decent cookbook or recipe collection, start with the basics. Some of my favorites are listed here (this is in no way, shape, or form a complete list).

Cookbooks:

- *American Heart Association Meals in Minutes Cookbook*
- *American Diabetes Association Great Recipes for You and Your Family*
- *Lickety Split Meals for Health Conscious People on the Go!* by Zonya Foco
- *Secrets of Feeding a Healthy Family* by Ellyn Satter
- *The Five in Ten Cookbook: Five Ingredients in Ten Minutes or Less* by Paula Hamilton

Magazines:

- *Taste of Home* and *Taste of Home's Light and Tasty* (filled with reader tips and recipes and *no* advertising!)
- *Cooking Light* (has a gourmet flare and great articles about wellness and exercise, too)
- *Eating Well* (in addition to recipes, contains articles on hot nutrition topics)

Websites:

- www.allrecipes.com
- www.epicurious.com/recipes
- www.allfood.com (check out the "minutemeals" section)
- www.mealsmatter.org (free registration gains access to a variety of meal-planning tools)

Eventually, you will develop a set of core recipes you can use over and over and tailor to your schedule, tastes, budget, and weekly bargains.

Experienced and novice cooks beware—don't be a slave to recipe modifications! In terms of health and sanity, it's more effective to consider *why* and *how much* you're eating than try to make every recipe you use conform to rigorous health standards.

If your all-time favorite dish is fried chicken, you may or may not enjoy a corn-flake crusted version of the bird. That's okay. If nothing but the original will do, enjoy fried chicken a little less frequently, and when you do, pair it with lower-fat side dishes such as cooked vegetables and fresh fruit. That makes sense not only for health reasons but also because it *tastes* good, and the number one reason people choose foods is taste! If you eat a whole bunch of low-fat, low-salt, sugar-free food, you may satisfy your immediate hunger, but your taste buds (your appetite) will still be hankering for more! So do yourself and your family a favor, and treat recipes with respect. Some of them lend themselves well to modification, and others are best left alone.

The following suggestions provide some *options* for altering recipes. Try a few of them, choose your favorites, and forget about the rest.

Baker's Corner

This is one area in which it pays to be cautious about recipe modification. Although cooking is an art that embraces all kinds of variations, baking tends to be more like a science. Small changes in ingredients often produce drastic changes in the finished product's taste and appearance, much to the chagrin of the health-conscious baker and his or her family members. Each ingredient in a baked good performs a vital function. Fat, for example, adds moisture and holds air in baked goods so that the final product is tender and light. Sugar provides bulk and tenderness and contributes to the nicely browned appearance of many baked goods. These are the two ingredients with which home bakers are most likely to tinker, so let's start there.

Reducing Sugar in Recipes

In many recipes, the sugar can be reduced by at least one-fourth without significantly affecting the final product. This is especially true of fruit-based pies, crisps, cobblers, and crumbles. You might grow to enjoy the flavor of a tart apple crisp even more so than overly sweet store-bought apple pies. If you find that reducing the sugar produces an unacceptable product, stick with your tried-and-true recipe and serve smaller portions. You might consume fewer calories by reducing portions than by modifying the recipe but eating a huge helping because it's "healthy."

note

Many people are experimenting with the array of artificial sweeteners on the market for their baking needs. You're welcome to try them, but beware that not all of them can be used at high temperatures, and they don't always measure cup for cup with sugar. They also tend to produce a slight aftertaste, which bothers some people and suits others just fine. The expense may also lead you to consider just eating smaller portions of baked goods made with the real stuff.

A few more pointers for reducing sugar in recipes:

- When decreasing sugar in cakes, use a smaller pan (use an 8-inch instead of a 9-inch pan)
- If reducing sugar for a cake, decrease the baking time by 10 minutes or more.
- For fruit-based desserts that call for large quantities of sugar, toss fruit with a few tablespoons of sugar, a bit of lemon juice, extra cinnamon or nutmeg, and a tablespoon or two of flour for thickener.

Reducing and Otherwise Altering the Fat in Baked Goods

As discussed previously, fat performs some vital functions in baked goods, so your safest bet is to make small changes and leave a little fat in the recipe:

- Substitute unsweetened applesauce or fruit purees for one-fourth up to one-half of the butter, shortening, or oil in cake, cookie, and quick bread recipes.
- Reduce the amount of ingredients such as nuts, coconut, and chocolate chips by one-third to one-half without causing a loss of flavor; try toasting chopped nuts to enhance the flavor and use less; use mini chocolate chips.
- If a recipe calls for shortening, which tends to contain a hefty amount of trans fat, try using a trans fat-free version. Read labels and follow directions on the package when substituting.
- It isn't usually wise to use a reduced-calorie butter or margarine in baking unless the label specifically states so. Most of these products have a high water content that changes their baking properties.

Adding Nutritional Value to Baked Goods

Registered dietitians are always looking for ways to improve the nutritional value of recipes. If it doesn't make a huge difference in quality, why not? Test the waters with these simple tips:

- Try substituting whole-wheat pastry flour for part or all of the all-purpose flour in recipes. Its light texture and whole-grain goodness makes it an ideal stand-in for all-purpose flour.
- If you can't find whole-wheat pastry flour, substitute regular whole-wheat flour for up to one-half of the all-purpose flour in recipes.
- Add extra dried, fresh, or frozen fruits to traditional recipes—extra berries in muffins; raisins or chopped dried plums in zucchini bread, banana bread, oatmeal cookies, or carrot cake; use mashed banana in cookie, muffin, and quick bread recipes for some of the fat.

Substitutes for Everyday Cooking

You've probably figured out by now that I'm not a fan of modifying your favorite recipes into oblivion. But with all kinds of products available, you might just find some that taste good to you and your family, and that help reduce the calories, fat, saturated fat, or anything else that concerns you. The suggestions in Table 9.2 can provide a few starting points.

TABLE 9.2   Painless Substitutions

Instead of...	Try...
Sour cream	Fat-free or low-fat sour cream, plain low-fat yogurt, or home-made yogurt cheese (see recipe earlier in the chapter).
Ricotta cheese	Low-fat or nonfat cottage cheese (or reduced-fat ricotta).
Whole milk	Skim, 1/2%, 1%, or 2% milk; nonfat dry milk; low-fat butter-milk; or evaporated skim milk, depending on use in recipe.
Heavy cream	Evaporated skim milk.
Butter or margarine	In cooking, simply reduce the amount (that is, sauté onions in a tablespoon of butter instead of 1/4 cup). Use a vegetable oil if possible (canola is a good choice for baking) or look for trans fat-free margarines and shortenings.
Regular salad dressing	Low-fat or fat-free dressings; low-fat yogurt, herbs, and spices; balsamic vinegar, olive oil, salt, and pepper; homemade creamy dressing using buttermilk, salt and pepper, and any other dried herbs. Dilute creamy bottled dressings with a little water.
Regular mayonnaise	Low-fat or fat-free mayonnaise, low-fat plain yogurt.
Baking chocolate (1 oz.)	Cocoa (3 T cocoa + 1 T trans fat-free margarine).
Cream cheese	Light or nonfat cream cheese, homemade yogurt cheese (see recipe earlier in the chapter).
Chopped nuts	Substitute crunchy nugget-type cereal for some of the nuts and/or reduce the amount of chopped nuts; toasting the nuts briefly in a nonstick skillet over medium heat brings out the flavor.
Whole egg	Egg substitute (1/4 cup) or 2 egg whites.
Sauté in oil or butter	Sauté in nonstick skillet with nonstick spray or a smaller amount of monounsaturated oil such as olive or canola.

THE ABSOLUTE MINIMUM

- Keep food out of the Danger Zone—40° to 140° F.
- Cook foods to the proper temperatures.
- Wash your hands frequently.
- Plan a few meals and prepare your kitchen by getting rid of the junk and organizing what you have left.
- Familiarize yourself with common cooking terms.
- Experiment with herbs, spices, and unexpected flavor combinations.
- Modify recipes if you want, but don't go overboard—enjoy your food!

IN THIS CHAPTER

- Rediscover your body's need to be active

- Learn how small steps lead to big improve-
ments

- Become more active in a way that is safe and
fun for you

- Prevent injuries with proper techniques, progression, and preparation

- Don't get derailed—know when and how you
can treat your own injuries, and when you
need professional help

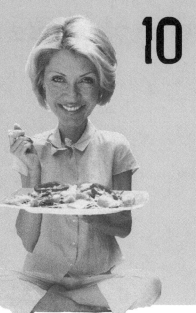

10

FITNESS FOR EVERY BODY

Why fitness for every body? Is this whole exercise thing really all that important? Can't you just watch what you eat and be healthy and forget about it? Well, you can, but the real question is why would you want to do that? Becoming more physically active has the potential to influence every area of your life. Think about it. Active people are better able to manage life challenges, achieve and maintain healthy body weights, and stay well throughout their lives than inactive people. They miss fewer days of work, get sick less often, and have more energy and vitality than their sedentary counterparts. An active lifestyle is within your reach, and you don't have to be an athlete or spend hours in a gym to achieve it. You do need to evaluate how activity will fit into your life, find activities that you enjoy, and go about it slowly and consistently. This chapter prepares you to do just that!

Ditch the Excuses and Make It Work for *You*

If you have always associated physical activity with pain, injury, inadequacy, and drudgery, it's time for a fresh approach. Human bodies were made to move! Whether you are small or large, lean or fat, short or tall, young or old, your body has an inherent need to be active every day. Being active can take as many different forms as there are people on the planet. For recreational and competitive athletes, it involves planned exercise to reach specific training goals; for families, it can include after-dinner walks and trips to a park on the weekends; for busy executives, exercise is an invaluable stress management tool. If you ask active people what keeps them motivated, you'll get a myriad of responses, but each one of them has found a reason (or many reasons!) to make physical activity a priority in his or her life. Your mission is to find out what motivates you.

People have all kinds of reasons for *not* being active. "Exercise is for jocks. I've never been an athlete, and I don't plan on becoming one," or "I exercised when I was younger, but I have a family, a stressful job, and more responsibility now. I just don't have time," or "I know I should exercise, but I don't know how. I want to do it right if I'm going to do it at all." Guess what? You can lead an active lifestyle even if you hate structured exercise, have an endless to-do list, and/or have never had formal training in planning an exercise program.

"Exercise is for jocks."

So you're never going to enter an Olympic competition—that's not an excuse to avoid activity altogether! What did you enjoy doing as a child? Did you like to dance? Play in the yard? Ride your bike? Go swimming? One of the most powerful ways to foster an active lifestyle is to seek out activities you actually enjoy. Don't wait for the perfect time or body weight, because there are no such things. Look for classes at the local college, walking clubs, exercise partners, swimming programs, or anything else that sounds interesting. If you have *never* enjoyed activity, now is the time for some personal exploration. Forget rules about how much, what kind, and how often you need to exercise; concentrate on incorporating activities that bring you joy.

"I don't have the time."

Sorry, but no deal. Everyone has 24 hours a day, and it's up to you to make activity a priority. Some of the most influential (and time pressed) people in the world are also devoted exercisers. It doesn't take hours in a gym, or even 30 minutes at one time. You can accumulate chunks of activity over the course of the day and have a positive impact on your overall health. Aim for 10 minutes a day at first. That's it. 10 minutes. You'll feel so good that you might just want to try 15 or 20 minutes next month. Your energy levels will increase, and you will be better able to fulfill your other responsibilities—how's that for payoff?

"I don't know how."

Don't get paralyzed by the details—it doesn't take a degree in fitness to be more active. Sure, after you've built a solid foundation, you might want to increase your exercise know-how, but don't wait till then to start moving. Can you walk? Swim? Bike? Jump up and down? Hula hoop? Dance? Play volleyball? Sit in a chair and move your arms? Then you can lead a more active lifestyle. You'll learn more detail about the what and how of exercise in Chapter 11, "Cardiovascular Training—The Foundation of an Exercise Program" and Chapter 12, "Strength Training 101," if you care to. For now, don't worry about doing it "right" and just start doing it!

Use the following exercise to help determine your motivational style and choose activities that reflect your style:

- Task—If you are task oriented, you enjoy accomplishment, structure, and personal improvement. You might enjoy solitary pursuits such as walking, running, lifting weights, cycling, paddling (kayaking), or hiking. It also helps to work with a fitness professional to design a program that enables you to see and record your progress.

- Social—If you are socially oriented, you enjoy participating in anything that involves other people. Try noon walks with co-workers, group exercise sessions at a local fitness center, or joining a cycling or walking club. Most cities offer group training programs for local long-distance running and walking events—check it out!

- Competitive—If you enjoy a good competition, choose activities that allow you to test your skills against others'. You may enjoy competitive sports such as basketball, racquetball, volleyball, and tennis. Training for an event can also provide the incentive you need to be consistent with activity. Look for local walks and runs, or find an event that supports a charity, research, or reputable organization.

- Extrinsic—If you are extrinsically motivated, tangible rewards and recognition are important to you. Working with a personal trainer or in a structured program may be a good way for you to get the recognition you need. You also need to pay special attention to rewarding yourself for your accomplishments—refer to the section "Smart Goals" in Chapter 2, "The Stages of Change—What to Expect," for a refresher course on developing appropriate rewards.

When it's time for you to actually hit the pavement, take note of the positive effects activity has on your life. Make a list, post it where you can see it every morning, and add to it as you become more fit. Your list might look something like the one shown in Figure 10.1.

FIGURE 10.1

The personal benefits of physical activity.

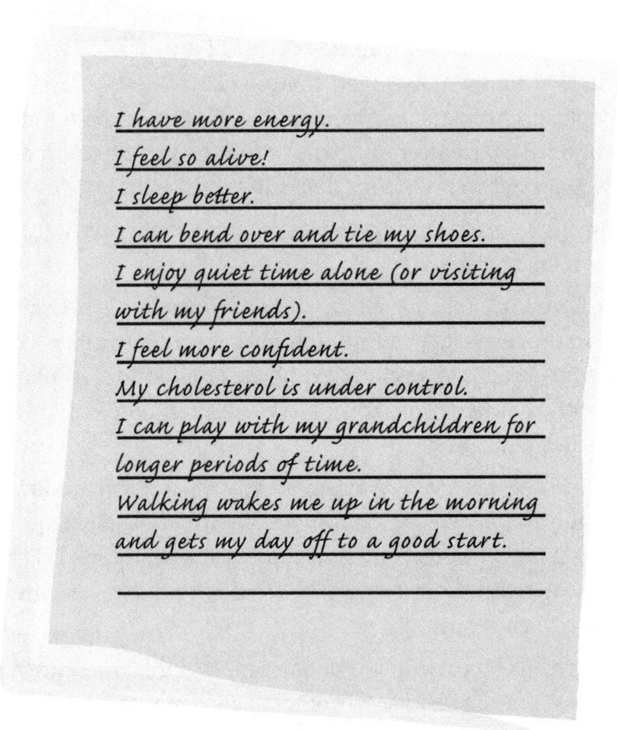

> *I have more energy.*
> *I feel so alive!*
> *I sleep better.*
> *I can bend over and tie my shoes.*
> *I enjoy quiet time alone (or visiting with my friends).*
> *I feel more confident.*
> *My cholesterol is under control.*
> *I can play with my grandchildren for longer periods of time.*
> *Walking wakes me up in the morning and gets my day off to a good start.*

What's on your list? Create one now and add to it as you go!

Make Your Mantra "Move More"

Before you jump into a structured exercise program, concentrate on increasing everyday movement, or lifestyle activity. It sounds so simple, doesn't it? You've probably heard it a hundred times before, but it's time to translate your *knowledge* into physical *action*. Many people who don't get the results they want from their exercise programs fail to lead active lives *outside* planned exercise. You have 168 hours each week, and even three hours of vigorous activity (although beneficial in many ways) is not enough to balance 165 sedentary hours.

Unfortunately, most of us live in an environment that is designed to minimize energy expenditure of any kind. Don't underestimate the impact of this environment. Think about the number of tools, devices, appliances, and other gadgets you use regularly that decrease the amount of physical energy you must expend:

- Riding lawn mowers
- Dishwashers
- Pay-at-the-pump gas stations
- Escalators and elevators
- Garage door openers
- Cell phones
- Automobiles
- Automatic locks, windows, and transmissions *in* your car!
- Internet shopping
- Email/voice mail
- Washer/dryer
- Electric mixer
- Drive-thru restaurants, banks, laundromats
- Automatic doors

note

If you find it difficult to move, work with a certified fitness instructor or physical therapist to develop solutions that make sense given your needs and physical abilities. Water aerobics courses are wonderful opportunities for people who have joint pain or who are uncomfortable or unable to move on land. Check out your local YMCA for resources in your area.

Can you think of others? It's easy to see how succumbing to the culture of inactivity can sideline your best intentions to lead a healthier lifestyle. Now's the time to break the mold! Use Figure 10.2 to brainstorm ways to become a little more active each day.

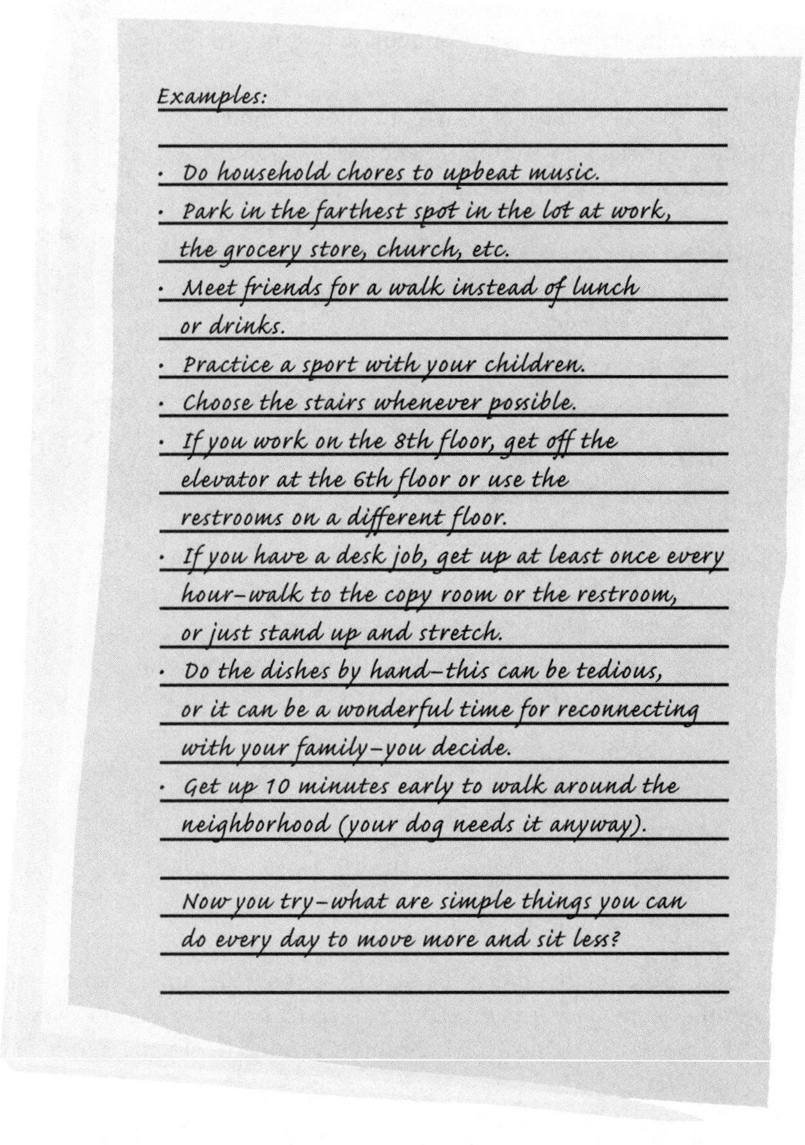

FIGURE 10.2
Find ways to
move more
each day.

Examples:

- *Do household chores to upbeat music.*
- *Park in the farthest spot in the lot at work,*
  the grocery store, church, etc.
- *Meet friends for a walk instead of lunch*
  or drinks.
- *Practice a sport with your children.*
- *Choose the stairs whenever possible.*
- *If you work on the 8th floor, get off the*
  elevator at the 6th floor or use the
  restrooms on a different floor.
- *If you have a desk job, get up at least once every*
  hour—walk to the copy room or the restroom,
  or just stand up and stretch.
- *Do the dishes by hand—this can be tedious,*
  or it can be a wonderful time for reconnecting
  with your family—you decide.
- *Get up 10 minutes early to walk around the*
  neighborhood (your dog needs it anyway).

Now you try—what are simple things you can
do every day to move more and sit less?

Many fitness-oriented New Year's resolutions are sidelined because experience fails to meet expectation. Change does not come easily, and it's not always a comfortable process. If you're making a commitment to a physically active lifestyle, go into it with eyes wide open to ensure that you have staying power. Understand and expect some or all of the following, and you'll avoid becoming a fitness dropout:

- Discomfort—If it's been a long time since you asked your body to move, expect a little flack from your muscles and joints. This doesn't usually last forever, but it can be discouraging for the novice exerciser. If you try a new activity and you're a little sore the next day, congratulate yourself—you've challenged your muscles, and they will respond by becoming stronger.

caution

This is *not* a recommendation to endure sharp or debilitating pain. This kind of pain is your body's way of preventing damage and further harm—respect it by discontinuing or modifying the activity in question.

- "Off" days—You won't always feel like getting up and moving, but you will inevitably feel better if you do it. Plenty of regular exercisers get out for their walks, runs, and rides even when they don't particularly want to, and they rarely regret it. How many things do you do every day that you don't feel like doing because the benefits you gain (or consequences you avoid) outweigh the associated costs? Physical activity is an investment in your life and the lives of those you love—start making deposits today!

note

If you're sick or exhausted, it is helpful to take a rest day or two (or more if needed). Rest is the body's way of healing, renewing energy stores, and keeping you fresh, and is an essential component of any exercise program.

- Plateaus—The pesky plateau can be enough to put anyone over the edge, but those who've stayed the course know plateaus aren't necessarily a bad thing. If you're on your way to a healthier body weight, a plateau is a sign that you've adjusted to new ways of eating and a new level of activity. Bask in the glory of a changed life! Focus on maintenance for a month or more and then evaluate whether you are ready to make additional changes. If you're involved in a planned exercise program and you've reached a plateau in strength or endurance or any other measure of fitness, work with a fitness professional to determine how to proceed. It's impossible to continue to improve indefinitely, and it helps to have an unbiased opinion about your exercise program from an expert.

Okay, you've just had a healthy dose of reality, and if you can swallow that, you're ready to move on. The following guidelines are designed to keep you safe and sane as you're exploring new territory in physical activity.

Injury Prevention and Damage Control

One of the most frustrating experiences for an active person is injury. Bad news first—injury has the potential to derail even the most dedicated of exercisers, and sometimes, end activity all together. The upside is that most injuries can be prevented by being mindful of some simple strategies in the following section. If you do become injured, you may be able to treat yourself with a little guidance, but when in doubt, see a physician for specific treatment recommendations. Pay attention to your body and listen to early warning signs (recurring aches and pains, swelling, inflammation, and so on) to avoid the hassle, headache, and pain of serious injury.

Warming Up, Cooling Down, and Getting Limber

The purpose of a warmup is to prepare your body for the real work. Compare it to preheating your oven—you wouldn't just throw that banana bread batter in a cold oven, turn it on, and expect an award-winning loaf, would you? Warming up allows your body temperature to increase slightly, loosens your joints and muscles, allows your heart and lungs to operate efficiently, reduces your risk of injury, and mentally helps prepare you for the exercise.

The key to a proper warmup is to take it nice and easy. The intensity during warmup should be light—you don't want to be huffing and puffing in the first 30 seconds. Walking and easy cycling are excellent choices. The goal is to elevate your heart and breathing rate slightly, and maybe even (gasp!) start to sweat a little. You're the best judge as to how long you should warm up. Some people are raring to go after a couple of minutes; others like to ease into their workout after 5 to 10 minutes of warming up. Listen to your body and respond appropriately.

Now let's assume that you're approaching the end of your workout. You're breathing hard, pouring sweat, and feeling amazing, but don't stop now! A 3- to 10-minute cool down allows your heart rate, blood pressure, and body temperature to gradually return to a pre-exercise condition. The cool down should mimic your warmup—keep performing your activity, but bring the intensity back down slowly until you feel ready to come to a complete stop.

Theories on stretching techniques abound, but the following guidelines hold true regardless of the specifics:

- Stretch *after* your warm up or *after* your entire exercise session to avoid injury caused by pulling cold, tight muscles.
- Remember to breathe. Inhale and exhale fully and deeply to relax your muscles and increase your range of motion.
- Stretch only to the point of mild tension or discomfort. If it hurts, stop—you may be performing the movement incorrectly or too intensely for your current level of flexibility.
- Avoid locking your joints—keep your knees and elbows slightly bent to prevent injury.
- Stretch with slow, controlled movements and hold the stretch for at least 10 to 15 seconds; avoid jerking or bouncing.

Are you ready to give it a shot? Remember to warm up first, and then try some or all of the exercises illustrated in the following sections.

Arm Circles

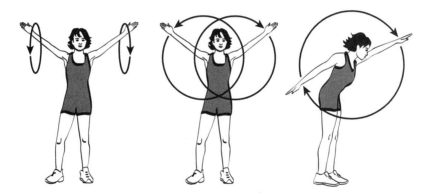

1. Stand with your feet apart, slightly wider than shoulder width, knees slightly bent, and arms at your side.
2. On each of the following arm stretches, swing your arms slowly with large, sweeping circles. Swing your arms from the shoulders, and keep your elbows straight but not locked.
   - Inward circles—Swing your arms inward, crossing in front of your body, moving upward, and over your head; repeat 10–15 times.
   - Outward circles—Swing your arms outward, crossing in front of your body, moving upward and over your head; repeat 10–15 times.

- Forward circles—Swing your arms alternately forward, with large sweeping circles, as if swimming. Count one complete circle with the left and right arm as one repetition; repeat 10–15 times.

- Backward circles—Swing your arms alternately backward, with large sweeping circles. Count one complete circle with the left and right arm as one repetition; repeat 10–15 times.

Shoulder Stretch

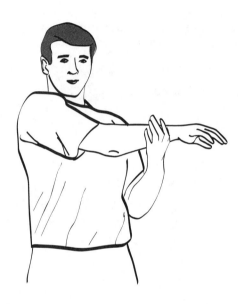

1. Stand or sit with your right arm across your chest.

2. Grasp your arm just above or below the elbow with your left hand.

3. Gently pull your right arm farther across your chest with your left hand.

4. Do not rotate your trunk in the direction of the stretch.

5. Hold for 10–30 seconds.

6. Repeat with your left arm, relax, and repeat 2–3 times with each arm.

Triceps Stretch (for the Back of Your Upper Arms)

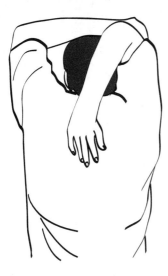

1. Standing or sitting, raise your right arm over your head.
2. Bend at the elbow and place your right hand on your back between your shoulder blades.
3. Grasp your right elbow with your left hand.
4. Gently pull your right elbow behind your head and downward.
5. Hold for 10–30 seconds.
6. Repeat with your left arm, relax, and repeat 2–3 times with each arm.

Side Stretch

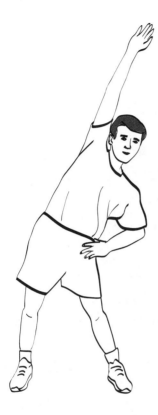

1. Stand with your feet apart, slightly wider than shoulder width, knees slightly bent, and toes pointing straight ahead.

2. Place your left hand on your left hip for support.

3. Lift your right arm up in line with your right ear and reach upward as high as possible.

4. Continue the stretch by arching your torso farther to the left. Be sure to stretch from the side and not twist at the waist.

5. Hold for 10–30 seconds.

6. Return your arms to side and repeat with your left arm overhead, relax, and repeat 2–3 times with each arm.

Hip Twist and Gluteal (Buttocks) Stretch

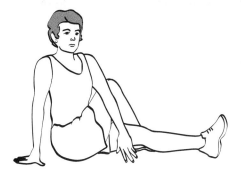

1. Sitting with your legs straight and upper body nearly vertical, place your right foot on the left side of your left knee.
2. Place the back of your left elbow on right side of your right knee, which is now bent.
3. Stabilize your upper body with your right hand placed 6–12 inches behind your right hip.
4. Gently push your right knee to the left with your left elbow while turning your shoulders and head to the right as far as possible.
5. Hold for 10–30 seconds.
6. Repeat with your left leg, relax, and repeat 2–3 times for each side.

Lower Back and Gluteal Stretch

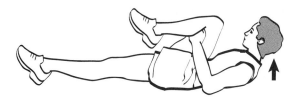

1. Lie on your back while pressing your lower back to the floor with both legs extended.
2. Bend your left knee, grasp behind your knee, and pull it toward your chest, while keeping your head on the floor.
3. Hold for 10–30 seconds; then curl your shoulders and lift your head and shoulders toward your knee.

4. Hold for 10 seconds.

5. Lower your shoulders, and then lower your left leg back to the floor and repeat with your right leg. Relax, and repeat 2–3 times for each leg.

Hamstring Stretch (for the Back of Your Upper Legs)

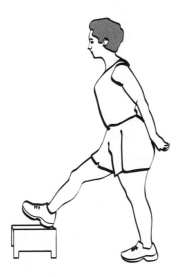

1. Stand with one foot propped up off the ground with your toes pointed up while the other leg is slightly bent and facing forward.

2. Keep your back straight (flat) and lean forward from the hips.

3. Hold stretch for 10–30 seconds.

4. Alternate legs, relax, and repeat 2–3 times for each leg.

Quadriceps Stretch (for the Front of Your Thighs)

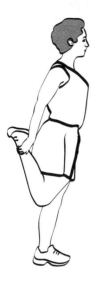

1. Stand on your left leg, holding onto a wall or fixed object with your left hand.

2. Bend your right knee and grasp your right ankle with your right hand, knee pointing down.

3. Slowly pull your right heel toward your buttocks. Do not pull on your ankle so hard that you feel pain or discomfort in the knee.

4. Keep your back straight and stand tall.

5. Hold for 10–30 seconds.

6. Repeat with your left leg, relax, and repeat 2–3 times for each leg.

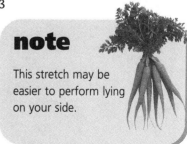

note

This stretch may be easier to perform lying on your side.

Groin Stretch

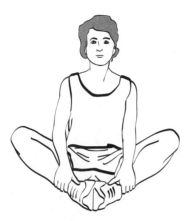

1. Sitting with your upper body nearly vertical and legs straight, bend both knees as the soles of your feet come together.

2. Grasp your ankles and pull your feet toward your body.

3. Place your hands on your feet and elbows on your thighs.

4. While keeping your back straight, pull your torso slightly forward as your elbows push your thighs down.

5. Hold for 10–30 seconds, relax, and repeat 2–3 times.

Gastrocnemius and Soleus Stretch (for the Backs of Your Lower Legs)

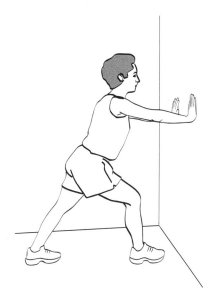

1. Stand facing a wall or other solid support. Place your outstretched hands or forearms on the wall.
2. Place your left leg behind your right leg, keeping your left leg straight.
3. Slowly move your hips and upper torso forward, keeping your back straight and the heel of your left foot on the ground (gastrocnemius stretch).
4. Hold stretch for 10–30 seconds.
5. Slowly begin to lower your body a few inches by bending your left knee and keeping the heel of both feet on ground (soleus stretch).
6. Hold for 10–30 seconds.
7. Repeat with the right leg behind the left, relax, and repeat 2–3 times for each leg.

Dress for Success—Choosing Shoes and Clothing for Maximum Comfort and Safety

The way you dress can have a significant impact on the quality of your workout, so don't skip this section in the name of speed! Nothing is worse than getting mentally prepared for exercise, and then discovering after you're outside or at the gym that your shoes are uncomfortable or you're not dressed appropriately. And although the importance of proper clothing varies depending on the activity you choose, most everyone needs a comfortable pair of shoes. The following guidelines can help you choose the best shoe for your needs:

- Try to find a shoe store that measures your feet. Many people discover that they are one-half to one full size bigger or smaller than expected!

- Because your feet expand while you run or walk, shop late in the day when your feet are at their widest and longest.

- Leave a thumb's width of room above your toes. Your toes should be able to move freely in the shoe.

- Your heel should be secure during all movement. If it slips up and down or side to side, the shoe is not giving enough support to your ankle and knee joints, and you could be inviting injury.

- Look for shoes with flared heels (wider where the base makes contact with the ground than with your foot). This is especially important if you plan on running or jogging, because it helps dissipate the impact over a larger surface area.

- Ask the salesperson if you can take the shoes for a little test run or walk on the sidewalk or in the mall concourse.

- Most running shoes make excellent walking shoes, too.

- Excessive wear compacts the cushioning material in shoes. If you plan to exercise most days of the week, you should probably replace your shoes every three to six months.

- It sounds obvious, but don't buy a shoe unless it's comfortable! You can get expert recommendations on the perfect shoe for your foot type and mode of exercise, but if it doesn't feel good, forget it!

After you have happy feet, you can move on to the rest of your body. If you choose to exercise outside, your clothing plays a huge role in your overall success. For both warm and cold weather activities, you'll want to wear a base layer of clothing that lets your skin breathe. The best materials are synthetic blends (*not* cotton), such as polypropylene, that actually wick away moisture and help sweat evaporate more quickly. You can find shorts, shirts, socks, and even underwear made from this kind of material at almost any department or sporting goods store, and you don't have to pay an arm and a leg to get it.

For cold weather activities, you'll need to add one or more layers on top of the breathable material to stay comfortable. Start with a light insulating layer made of some type of fleece, then add a wind resistant layer if it's very cold. Remember to cover your head and extremities as well, preferably with hats and gloves or mittens made of the same light synthetic material as your base layer. You can always remove clothing if you get too warm during the activity.

The heat index and wind chill can wreak havoc on your outdoor exercise plans. Use Figures 10.3 and 10.4 to help you prepare for the conditions appropriately.

tip

If you're going for a run or walk in cold weather, you should feel a little chilly when you first step outside. If you feel toasty and warm right out of the house, you're probably overdressed.

FIGURE 10.3

How cold does it feel when the wind blows?

Wind Chill Chart

Frostbite Times

☐ 30 minutes

☐ 10 minutes

☐ 5 minutes

Wind (mph)	Temperature (°F)								
Calm	40	30	20	10	0	-10	-20	-30	-40
5	36	25	13	1	-11	-22	-34	-46	-57
10	34	21	9	-4	-16	-28	-41	-53	-66
15	32	19	6	-7	-19	-32	-45	-58	-71
20	30	17	4	-9	-22	-35	-48	-61	-74
25	29	16	3	-11	-24	-37	-51	-64	-78
30	28	15	1	-12	-26	-39	-53	-67	-80
35	28	14	0	-14	-27	-41	-55	-69	-82
40	27	13	-1	-15	-29	-43	-57	-71	-84
45	26	12	-2	-16	-30	-44	-58	-72	-86
50	26	12	-3	-17	-31	-45	-60	-74	-88
55	25	11	-3	-18	-32	-46	-61	-75	-89
60	25	10	-4	-19	-33	-48	-62	-76	-91

While we're talking about dressing for the weather, let's address one other safety issue for exercise in the great outdoors—heat illness.

FIGURE 10.4

How hot does it feel when the humidity rises?

Apparent Temperature Chart

Air Temperature (°F)

	0	**5**	**10**	**15**	**20**	**25**	**30**	**35**	**40**	**45**	**50**	**55**	**60**	**65**	**70**	**75**	**80**	**85**	**90**	**95**	**100**
120	108	112	117	124	131	135															
115	104	107	110	116	120	128	138														
110	99	102	105	108	112	117	123	130	139												
105	95	98	100	102	105	108	113	117	122	130	140	155									
100	91	93	95	97	98	102	104	107	110	115	120	126	132	138							
95	86	88	89	91	93	95	98	100	104	106	109	113	119	124	130	136	142	147	153	155	
90	82	84	85	86	87	88	90	91	92	95	97	98	100	103	106	110	114	117	121	125	130
85	77	78	80	81	82	83	84	85	86	87	87	89	90	92	94	96	97	100	102	105	108
80	73	74	75	76	77	78	78	79	79	80	81	82	83	84	85	86	87	88	88	90	92
75	69	70	70	71	71	72	73	74	74	75	75	76	76	76	77	77	77	78	78	79	80
70	65	65	66	66	67	67	68	68	68	68	69	69	70	70	70	71	71	72	72	73	73

Relative Humidity (%)

Caution: Fatigue possible with prolonged exposure and physical activity (80° to 89°F).

Extreme Caution: Sunstroke, Heat Cramps, or Heat Exhaustion possible with prolonged exposure and physical activity (90° to 104°F).

Danger: Sunstsroke, Heat Cramps, or Heat Exhaustion likely; Heatstroke possible with prolonged exposure and physical activity (105° to 129°F).

Extreme Danger: Heatstroke or Sunstroke imminent (130°F or more).

Heat and humidity cause the body to work much harder than usual. In very humid conditions, your body can't control core temperature efficiently because sweat doesn't evaporate from the skin. Exercising in hot, humid weather is of particular concern for children, the elderly, heavier people, and people who just plain sweat a lot. Use the following guidelines to prevent heat-related injury:

- Hydrate properly. Your thirst mechanism works well under normal circumstances, but it might not be able to keep pace in adverse conditions. Drink one to two cups of fluid at least 15 minutes before your activity and then drink one-half to one cup of fluid every 15 minutes during activity. You can even weigh yourself before and after exercise (in the nude) to be sure you didn't lose too much water weight. If your weight has dropped, you need to drink at least two cups of fluid for every pound you lost. If you're exercising for an hour or less, water will probably be just fine. If you're exercising longer than that, you may want to consider a sports beverage that can supply carbohydrate and replace electrolytes, such as sodium and potassium, that are lost through sweat.

- Let your body get acclimated to the weather before you attempt a full workout. In other words, if you've been exercising indoors all winter and into spring, don't jump into outdoor summer workouts until you've done some light activity outside regularly for at least a week.

▓ Avoid exercising in the heat of the day—from 10 a.m. to 3 p.m. in many areas. In other locations, the hottest time of day is as late as 4 p.m. Set your alarm a half-hour early, or recruit an exercise partner for a late evening session, just don't subject yourself to the punishing sun if possible!

▓ Wear light, breathable clothing.

▓ If you notice any of the following symptoms, stop exercising, get out of the sun, drink cool beverages, remove clothing, and apply ice packs if desired:

   ▓ Progressive weakness, reduced appetite

   ▓ Moist, clammy skin

   ▓ Rapid but weak pulse

▓ If any or all of the following occur, seek medical attention for heat stroke immediately:

   ▓ Dizziness, weakness, and confusion

   ▓ Loss of consciousness

   ▓ Elevated body temperature (105° F is not uncommon in people suffering from heat stroke)

   ▓ Flushed, hot, dry skin

The Importance of Progression

You can be dressed to the nines, warmed up, and stretched out, but if you jump into an activity that is too intense for your current fitness level, you're inviting pain at the least, and serious injury or even death at the worst. Are you paying attention now? *Progression* is the key to preventing all of this! It's amazing how many people ignore this simple concept and end up quitting their exercise programs because they just don't feel good, or they wind up with knee, foot, and various other problems. Any time you begin a new activity, take things slowly. Do a little bit at a time, and see how it affects your body. It's always best to err on the conservative side, so don't feel guilty because you can't do very much at first. Keep progression in mind no matter what activity you're performing.

Treating Injuries with R.I.C.E.

Sometimes people sustain injuries despite their best efforts to prevent them. The trick is to know when you can handle injuries on your own, and when you should seek medical treatment. If you experience any of the following symptoms, seek professional treatment as soon as possible:

- Shooting, sharp, or debilitating pain
- Soreness in muscles or joints that gets worse with time
- Excessive swelling, discoloration, numbness, or tingling
- If in doubt, check it out! (with your physician)

For minor aches and pains, the *R.I.C.E. principle* can be helpful. The key is to treat minor injuries as quickly as possible. If your knee is giving you a little trouble, don't try to tough it out and just keep walking or running on it. Many minor injuries become serious problems because people fail to listen to their bodies!

R = Rest

Rest the affected muscle group or body part to prevent further injury. Discontinue the movement or exercise until you're back to normal.

I = Ice

Ice constricts the blood vessels in the area of injury and helps minimize inflammation, swelling, and pain. Cover the entire area with an ice pack, zip-top bag filled with ice, or a bag of frozen peas or corn specially designated for this purpose (who knew vegetables were so versatile?). Your skin may feel a little uncomfortable at first, but you are not in any danger of frostbite (your body heat will melt the ice before it can cause any damage). If you are able, apply the cold pack for up to 20 to 30 minutes three to four times a day for the first two or three days.

C = Compression

Compression can be a little tricky for beginners, so use it only if you feel comfortable, or if you have a knowledgeable friend who can help. By compressing the injured area, you can limit swelling by pushing excess fluid out of the area and back into the circulation. Apply compression by wrapping the injured area with elastic wrap, starting at the location farthest from your heart. For example, if your wrist is injured, start wrapping closer to your fingers than to your arm. You can create a pumping action by wrapping a little more tightly as you begin, and easing up a bit as you finish the wrap. Be sure to avoid wrapping so tightly that you cut off the blood supply to the extremity—check your fingertips or toes by pressing them and then seeing whether the blood comes back quickly. If they stay white, or if they turn red or bluish purple, remove the wrap and try again!

E = Elevation

This is an easy one! If possible, elevate the injured area above the level of the heart so that gravity can help drain excess fluid.

THE ABSOLUTE MINIMUM

- Let go of excuses and find activities consistent with your personality and lifestyle.
- Find ways to move more and sit less each day.
- Expect a little discomfort as you become more active.
- Prevent injuries by dressing appropriately, warming up prior to activity, cooling down after activity, and preparing for weather conditions.
- Stretch muscles after you're warmed up or after your activity in a slow, controlled fashion.
- Progression is the key to preventing 95% of injuries!
- Treat minor injuries with rest, ice, compression, and elevation.

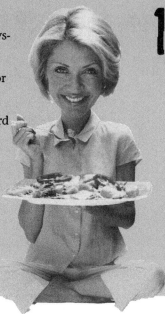

11

Cardiovascular Training—The Foundation of an Exercise Program

Cardiovascular training is the kind of training everyone visualizes when you mention "exercise." Cardiovascular training gets your heart pumping, your blood moving, your lungs heaving, and your body sweating. It has the potential to produce the "runner's high," be mildly pleasant, or be not much fun at all depending on how you approach it. The key, as emphasized in Chapter 10, "Fitness for Every Body," is to begin slowly, go at your own pace, and have fun with it. For those who appreciate a little structure, this chapter provides just that in the form of the *F.I.T.T. principle*, which stands for Frequency, Intensity, Time, and Type.

Cardiovascular Training—What Is It?

First, let's distinguish cardiovascular training from plain old physical activity. In Chapter 10, we sort of lumped it all together, but it's helpful to understand the uniqueness of cardiovascular training.

Physical activity really includes any type of bodily movement. It's not limited to planned sessions of activity and includes things such as walking to the corner store, parking farther away from building entrances, cleaning the house, raking leaves, walking up a flight of stairs, even making the bed in the morning. These types of movements definitely expend energy and are keys to a healthy lifestyle, but they may or may not challenge your cardiovascular system.

Cardiovascular training, on the other hand, is designed to do precisely that—improve your cardiovascular fitness by challenging your heart and lungs to work a little (or a lot) harder than usual for a specified amount of time. It's also sometimes referred to as aerobic exercise. Your options for cardiovascular training are limitless, but look for those that interest you in Figure 11.1.

If you're wondering why you need to incorporate cardiovascular training in addition to increasing daily activity, look no further! Cardiovascular training supplies a unique challenge to your cells, tissues, and systems that has been shown to improve all kinds of health parameters. For example, cardiovascular training increases your body's sensitivity to insulin, a hormone that gives blood glucose access to your cells. Once inside the cells, glucose can be used for energy. By improving insulin sensitivity, you can reduce your risk for developing diabetes, or reduce your need for medication and/or insulin if you already have diabetes. Ready for more? Take a look at this list of potential benefits from cardiovascular training:

- Decreases risk for cardiovascular disease
- Increases HDL (good) cholesterol
- Decreases risk for osteoporosis
- Improves sleeping patterns
- Promotes healthy body weight
- Lowers blood pressure
- Decreases risk for cancer
- Decreases risk for osteoarthritis
- Improves immune function
- Increases energy levels

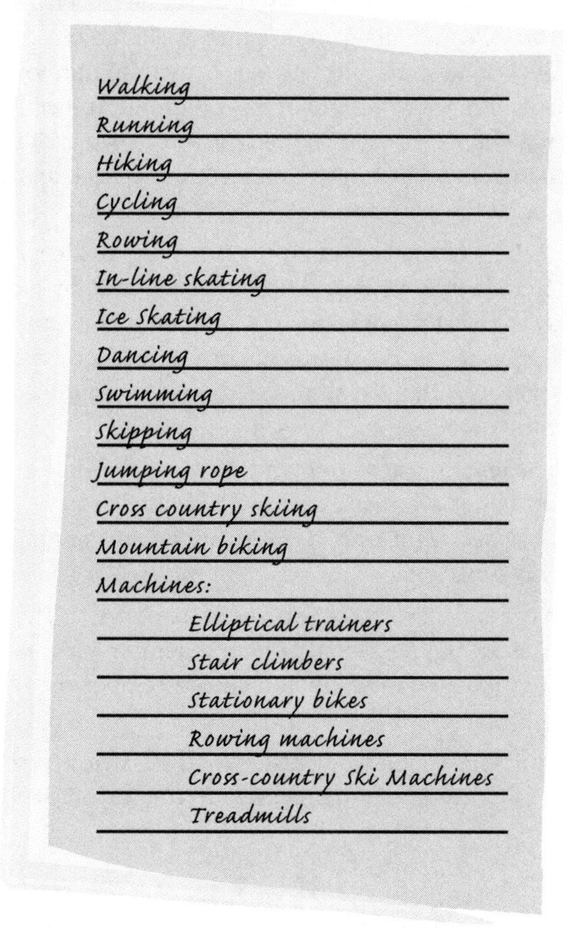

FIGURE 11.1

Cardiovascular training—pick one that works for you!

Walking

Running

Hiking

Cycling

Rowing

In-line skating

Ice Skating

Dancing

Swimming

Skipping

Jumping rope

Cross country skiing

Mountain biking

Machines:

Elliptical trainers

Stair climbers

Stationary bikes

Rowing machines

Cross-country Ski Machines

Treadmills

Sometimes it helps to put a human touch to the clinical benefits. Nellie has an amazing story about the power of exercise.

Patience and Persistence Pay Off (Nellie's Story)

Nellie (not her real name) had been on and off diets and exercise programs for most of her life. She had her first child at the age of 21 and struggled with her weight ever since, going on a total of 11 formal diet programs. She was hypnotized, had her ear stapled, participated in a supervised medical weight loss plan, and joined several well-known commercial weight loss programs. While she and her husband raised four children, she worked full time, went back to school to work on her degree, and continued to battle weight and health issues through it all. Nellie had just about given up when a close friend, Sandra (not her real name), encouraged her to join a 12-week lifestyle management program at NIFS. Sandra had had her own struggles with body weight and health but was convinced that together, she and Nellie could make it work with the help of this program. At first, Nellie resisted, but Sandra wouldn't take no for an answer. Pretty soon the two became regulars at the fitness center, working out together two to three times a week and attending educational sessions through the program.

It wasn't easy, especially in the beginning. "It was hell," Nellie remarked frankly. "I didn't know if I could do it. But I started feeling better, and my blood pressure was going down. I may even get to adjust my medications in a couple months." What was different about this program? "It was the first time I had combined nutrition with exercise. With every other diet plan, exercise was encouraged, but I got no formal support or instruction."

Nellie's advice for beginners: Know that "there are people who care, and you can make progress, but it's not overnight, and you have to be *patient*. I thought 'how long do I want to live and what kind of quality of life do I want to have?' and it kept me going. The key is *persistence*."

Nellie and Sandra are still close friends and exercise partners. They attend a weekly support group and share their experiences with other participants. Both of them believe that their mutual accountability is a crucial component in maintaining their new lifestyles.

Are you ready to quit reading and get outside for a brisk walk yet? Before you do, get a grasp on how to incorporate cardiovascular training efficiently with the F.I.T.T. principle.

F Is for Frequency—How Often Should You Train?

If you aren't good with numbers, think *regularly*. If you like to be a little more specific, experts suggest you aim for at least three and up to five or six days a week of cardiovascular training. Don't forget the concept of progression! If you're starting from scratch, try to work in one to two days of cardiovascular training per week. When you're comfortable with that much, you can build up to three, four, even five or six days per week.

note

It's fine to train up to six days a week, but be sure to take at least one full day of rest or very light activity so that your body has a chance to repair tissues and build up energy stores for the week ahead.

I Is for Intensity—How Hard Should You Train?

There are several ways to determine how hard you should be working when you engage in cardiovascular training. One is very specific and involves calculating a target heart rate range and then monitoring your heart rate during activity to determine whether you're "in the zone." You can get a rough estimate of this range by using the calculations shown in Figure 11.2, but because every person's needs are a little different, it's ideal to consult a health fitness professional to determine an appropriate target heart rate range for you. Figure 11.3 shows an example of calculating the target heart rate range.

Rating of Perceived Exertion

The other two ways to gauge your intensity are less scientific but more practical. One is called a *Rating of Perceived Exertion (RPE) scale* and involves subjectively rating your level of effort on a scale of 0 to 10. The nice thing about an RPE scale is that it accounts for differences in individual fitness levels, sick days, and off days instead of dogmatically dictating a number that may or may not be appropriate given the circumstances. Use Figure 11.4 to become familiar with the RPE scale.

Beginners can aim for exercising at the three to four rating (moderate to somewhat strong), whereas more advanced exercisers can strive for a rating of five to eight (strong to very strong). As you progress, activities that used to be difficult will likely become a little easier to perform. If you find that walking around your neighborhood no longer feels challenging, either try a new activity or walk more quickly so that your effort level stays around a three to four instead of dropping down to a one or two.

The Talk Test

Another practical method of determining whether you are exercising at an appropriate intensity is the *talk test*. The least scientific of the three methods, but definitely the most user friendly, the talk test involves a simple self-assessment during exercise. You should be able to hold a conversation with an exercise partner, a pet, or yourself (out loud) without too much difficulty. If you're huffing and puffing so much that you can't complete a sentence, try backing down the intensity a bit. On the other hand, if you can sing your favorite tune while exercising, you probably aren't working hard enough. Simple, but effective!

FIGURE 11.2

Take these steps
to determine
your target
heart rate
range.

Steps to determine your appropriate target heart rate range:

1. **Estimated Maximal Heart Rate** (220 - age) =

2. **Resting Heart Rate** for 3 days (taken first thing in the morning) and calculate the average:

   Day 1 _____ Day 2 _____ Day 3 _____   Average of 3 days = _____

3. Maximal Heart Rate minus Average Resting Heart Rate = **Heart Rate Reserve** (HRR)

   _____ – _____ = _____
      (#1)   (#2)

4. **Training Intensity Range** (Heart Rate Reserve x 50-85%):

   Easy

   (HRR x 0.50) _____ x 0.50 = _____ beats per minute
               (#3)

   (HRR x 0.65) _____ x 0.65 = _____ beats per minute
               (#3)

   Moderate

   (HRR x 0.65) _____ x 0.65 = _____ beats per minute
               (#3)

   (HRR x 0.75) _____ x 0.75 = _____ beats per minute
               (#3)

   Hard

   (HRR x 0.75) _____ x 0.75 = _____ beats per minute
               (#3)

   (HRR x 0.85) _____ x 0.85 = _____ beats per minute
               (#3)

5. Add the Average Resting Heart Rate to the Training Intensity Range to find your **Target Heart Rate Range.**

   Easy

   _____ + (_____ to _____) = _____ to _____ beats per minute
     (#2)   (50% to 65% from #4)

   Moderate

   _____ + (_____ to _____) = _____ to _____ beats per minute
     (#2)   (65% to 75% from #4)

   Hard

   _____ + (_____ to _____) = _____ to _____ beats per minute
     (#2)   (75% to 80% from #4)

FIGURE 11.3

Here is a hypo-
thetical
example.

For example, Susie is 45 years old:

1. **Estimated Maximal Heart Rate** (220 - age) = 175

2. **Resting Heart Rate** for 3 days (taken first thing in the morning) and calculate the average:

   Day 1 = 75   Day 2 = 72   Day 3 = 76

   Average of 3 days = $\dfrac{\text{(Day 1 + Day 2 + Day 3)}}{3}$ = $\dfrac{223}{3}$ **74 beats per minute**

3. Maximal Heart Rate minus Average Resting Heart Rate = **Heart Rate Reserve** (HRR)

   175 — 74 = **101 beats per minute**
   (From #1) (From #2)

4. **Training Intensity Range** (Heart Rate Reserve x 50-85%):

   Easy

   (HRR x 0.50) 101   x   0.50 = **51 beats per minute**
   (From #3)
   (HRR x 0.65) 101   x   0.65 = **66 beats per minute**
   (From #3)

   Moderate

   (HRR x 0.65) 101   x   0.65 = **66 beats per minute**
   (From #3)
   (HRR x 0.75) 101   x   0.75 = **76 beats per minute**
   (From #3)

   Hard

   (HRR x 0.75) 101   x   0.75 = **76 beats per minute**
   (From #3)
   (HRR x 0.85) 101   x   0.85 = **86 beats per minute**
   (From #3)

5. Add the Average Resting Heart Rate to the Training Intensity Range to find your **Target Heart Rate Range.**

Easy

74   +   (51 to 66)   =   **125 to 140** beats per minute
(From #2)   (50% to 65% from #4)

Moderate

74   +   (66 to 76)   =   **140 to 150** beats per minute
(From #2)   (65% to 75% from #4)

Hard

74   +   (76 to 86)   =   **150 to 160** beats per minute
(From #2)   (75% to 85% from #4)

FIGURE 11.4

Use the Rating of Perceived Exertion (RPE) scale to gauge how hard you're working during cardiovascular training.

Rating		Sample activities
0	Total rest	Watching TV
1	Very light	
2	Light	Riding a bicycle/brisk walking
3	Moderate	
4	Somewhat strong	
5	Strong	
6		
7	Very strong	Rollerblading
8		
9		
10	Maximum effort	All out sprinting

T Is for Time (or Duration)—How Long Should You Train?

Again, to put things in perspective, you'll get health benefits from even the smallest increases in physical activity and short bouts of cardiovascular training. However, to improve your cardiovascular fitness level, you'll want to eventually work your way up to 30 to 60 minutes of continuous cardiovascular training. Exercising for periods longer than 60 minutes can be beneficial if you're training for endurance events, and perhaps in weight management, but isn't necessary for general health and fitness. Once again, progression is key, so if you aren't yet comfortable with 30 minutes at one time, start with shorter bouts and just be consistent!

tip

If you've been sedentary for a long time, maybe your whole life, it would be reasonable, and perhaps most beneficial, to focus on increasing the duration of your workouts before even considering intensity. This minimizes your risk for injury and maximizes your level of enjoyment through the whole process. Even if you can only walk to your mailbox and back, you *can* succeed at cardiovascular training by respecting your body and its capabilities. Next week, add a few extra steps; the following week, another block. As they say, "slow and steady wins the race!"

T Is for Type of Activity—Which Exercises Are Right for You?

Choosing the right activity is crucial to your health, success, and motivation when it comes to cardiovascular training. Ask yourself a few questions so that you can find activities you will continue to enjoy for a lifetime:

- Is it fun? Will you really enjoy this activity? If you like to work alone, running or walking may best suit your needs. If you're a social butterfly, consider joining walking and running groups, swim clubs, or group fitness classes, or simply recruit an exercise buddy!

■ Is it convenient? Does the exercise require special equipment or facilities? If so, can you afford it? Do you travel frequently? Don't waste your money on a gym membership or fancy equipment if you prefer to exercise outside.

■ Does it fit into your schedule? Planning exercise into your day like any other important event is crucial. The goal is to find a time that works for *you*, whether in the morning, at lunch, or in the evening. Put it on your calendar so you're less likely to let exercise be "bumped" by other commitments.

note

There's no "correct" time of day to exercise, but many studies show that morning exercisers tend to be more successful with their programs. It isn't because of some metabolic advantage of working out early in the day but because morning exercisers tend to be the most *consistent* with their routines. If you find that other responsibilities are crowding your after-work or evening exercise sessions, try getting up early for a week and squeezing in a short routine before the day gets under way. You'll be glad you did! See the section "There Are No Excuses at 5:30 in the Morning" for inspiration.

There Are No Excuses at 5:30 in the Morning (Jill's Story)

It took Jill (not her real name) a lifetime of experiences, setbacks, successes, and personal growth to reach her current level of fitness and develop healthy attitudes and eating patterns. Jill was normal weight as a child until her parents divorced when she was seven years old. At that point, food started becoming an issue.

"By the time I was nine, I was definitely overweight. I turned to food because I knew it wouldn't go away. I found comfort in food when I came home to an empty house. It was very emotionally driven eating."

Jill had always been self-conscious about her body. Her weight went up and down, depending on life circumstances and her level of commitment to exercising. She became so committed, in fact, that her weight was driven unnaturally low for her height and body type. She knew that she had become obsessed when she found herself at the gym two times a day, and eventually sustained an injury that forced her to quit altogether. At that point, the pounds started creeping back on, and Jill found herself entangled in destructive behaviors and attitudes.

"I've always struggled with food and exercise. I was obsessive about the number...I ate or didn't eat based on my weight for the day."

A turning point came when Jill decided to join a 12-week lifestyle management program at NIFS that encourages participants to get back to basics with nutrition, exercise, and wellness.

"The class came at the right time for me. I had to ask for help, and I needed the support. I reintroduced fruits and vegetables, and it really helped to keep a food log and turn it in each week…I think I might have to work on my body image for a long time, but I know now what's reasonable and what isn't, and I'm working on it."

Jill no longer turns to food for emotional comfort, and she is a regular morning exerciser in the NIFS Fitness Center. She really enjoys the elliptical machines and has even begun incorporating "intervals" of high-intensity training into her 50-minute routine. She and her exercise buddy plan to up it to 60 minutes at the first of the year. How does she maintain motivation for her early morning workouts?

"The hardest part is actually physically getting up and putting your feet on the floor. After you've done that, the rest isn't so bad. It's hard to get up early, but you do it anyway. I feel so much better when I do, and you know, there are no excuses at 5:30 in the morning."

If you're brand new to cardiovascular training, choose an activity with which you feel comfortable and confident. Walking is one of the simplest ways to get started because you don't need much more than a decent pair of shoes and a safe place to walk. If you are uncomfortable walking outside, try mall walking. Many malls are teeming with walkers early in the morning before hard-core shopping gets underway. See Table 11.1 for a sample beginner's walking program.

TABLE 11.1   A Beginner's Walking Program

Week	Monday	Tuesday	Wednesday	Thursday	Friday	Saturday	Sunday	Total
1	10–20 min	REST	10–20 min	REST	REST	10–20 min	REST	30–60 min
2	15–20 min	REST	15–20 min	REST	REST	15–20 min	REST	45–60 min
3	20–25 min	REST	20–25 min	REST	REST	20–25 min	REST	60–75 min
4	20–30 min	REST	20–30 min	REST	REST	20–30 min	REST	60–90 min

If you enjoy walking, you might consider investing in a little device called a *pedometer*. A pedometer looks somewhat like a pager and can be fastened to the waist of your pants or skirt with a clip. Whenever you wear the pedometer, it tracks the number of steps you take with a small sensor that detects impact. Some pedometers can also provide information about time and distance, and even estimate calorie expenditure. Many walking programs encourage participants to aim for 10,000 steps a day. It's a fairly arbitrary way of encouraging people to walk approximately five miles each day, through both structured exercise and activities of daily living.

You might find that 10,000 steps is far beyond your reach at this point, and, if so, just start building on your daily average slowly and consistently. If you average 2,000 steps daily the first week you wear the pedometer, aim for 2,250 steps daily the second week. If that feels comfortable, shoot for 2,500 steps the following week, slowly working your way to 10,000 or more steps daily. The pedometer provides objective information about how much you're really moving each day and encourages you to take more walk breaks, go a little farther on your planned walks, and be less sedentary overall. Not a bad deal for such an unpretentious little tool!

note

Most people average 2,000 steps and 100 calories per mile; so walking 10,000 steps is the equivalent of five miles and 500 calories.

THE ABSOLUTE MINIMUM

- Cardiovascular training gets your heart, lungs, and blood pumping and is associated with numerous positive health effects—think of it as the "elixir" of good health!

- Choose activities you enjoy.

- Start small; if you're brand new to cardiovascular activity, try 5- or 10-minute chunks.

- Work your way up to 30 to 60 minutes of continuous cardiovascular activity most days of the week (three to five is a good average).

- Train at an intensity that feels challenging, but not overwhelming—use your target heart rate range, the RPE scale, or the talk test to monitor how hard you're working.

- Recruit a buddy and have fun!

- Discover why strength training matters

- Become familiar with strength training lingo

- Understand strength training techniques to keep you safe and sane

- Rediscover your major muscle groups and learn how to stimulate each of them with a balanced training program

- Dispel common myths about strength training

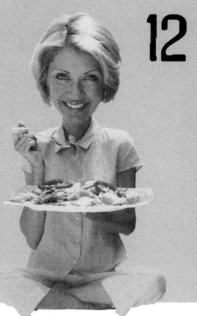

Strength Training 101

Strength training is the kind of training that requires your muscles to overcome some type of resistance, whether from your own body weight, hand-held weights, or special machines and equipment. It's a little more challenging for beginners, simply because it requires skills and movements with which you may be unfamiliar. Don't fret—you really can master strength training and start reaping the benefits with a little patience, practice, and time.

Why Bother?

Okay, you've read all about cardiovascular training and how great it is for your overall health, but why stop there? Strength training offers many unique benefits for people of all ages, abilities, and fitness levels.

During the first 30 years of life, strength and muscle mass increase steadily as you grow, but most people begin to lose muscle strength and mass beginning in their early thirties. Research shows that if you are sedentary after age 30, lean muscle mass deteriorates at a rate of approximately one-half percent per year. That's the equivalent of five to seven pounds of muscle every decade! In fact, the older you get, the more beneficial it is to incorporate strength training in your lifestyle. If you need a little more persuasion, read on!

Avoid Muscle Loss

Walking, running, cycling, and other aerobic activities are great for your heart and lungs, but they are limited in their ability to build and maintain your muscle mass. Results of strength training programs depend on genetics, nutrition, quality of training, and other factors, but most people can expect significant gains in muscle strength and endurance (see "Terms, Tips, and Tools of the Trade" later in this chapter) by training consistently (two or three times per week) in as little as two months.

Keep Metabolism Elevated

Muscle is a metabolically active tissue. A person who has more muscle tissue (lean body mass) burns more calories even at rest than someone with less muscle tissue. Without regular strength training, most people need fewer and fewer calories each year, but frequently find it difficult to eat less to adjust for the difference. Strength training can help prevent this gradual lowering of energy expenditure as you age.

Increase Bone Density

Osteoporosis is a debilitating disease in which bones become porous, spongy, and susceptible to fractures. Regular strength training has been shown to increase bone mineral density in just a few months and thus reduce the risk for osteoporosis. If you are deficient in dietary calcium (refer to Figure 4.5 on page 61), are thin-framed, female, of Asian decent, or have a family history of the disease, you are at even greater risk, so pumping some iron can be particularly helpful.

Reduce Body Fat

This point underscores the metabolic benefits of strength training. The more muscle mass you have, the more calories you burn. By eating and exercising consistently, and incorporating strength training, you will likely begin to lose body fat and build muscle mass. This sometimes means that the scale doesn't move much, but your clothes will probably fit differently, and you might notice changes in the way you look and feel. This illustrates why it is important to focus on measures other than body weight to track progress.

Terms, Tips, and Tools of the Trade

You need to be familiar with some key terms and concepts before you can jump into planning your own strength training program:

- *Muscle strength* is the ability of the muscles to contract maximally one time only—in other words, how much you can lift.
- *Muscle endurance* is the ability of the muscles to contract repeatedly—in other words, how many times you can lift a certain weight.
- *Concentric contraction* is the shortening of the muscle during a contraction and is typically the harder portion of the movement. For example, when doing a bicep curl, the concentric contraction occurs when your fist is moving toward your shoulder.
- *Eccentric contraction* is the lengthening of the muscle during a contraction and is typically the easier portion of the movement. The eccentric contraction of the bicep curl occurs when your arm is straightening.
- *Repetition (rep)*—One complete movement from start to finish.
- *Set*—A group of repetitions.

Any time you perform strength training, remember the following:

- Warm up—Three to five minutes of light aerobic exercise (walking, jogging, rowing, and so on) is an adequate warmup for strength training. Your warmup increases heart rate, blood flow, respiration rate, and deep muscle temperature, and may reduce your risk for injury.
- Breathe—Proper breathing techniques can help you stay safe and perhaps even perform more efficiently. Try to inhale on the easier portion of the movement (eccentric contraction) and exhale on the harder part (concentric contraction). If you forget which part is which, just don't hold your breath!

■ Exercise order—Begin strength training sessions with exercises that target the larger muscle groups and then move to the smaller ones. For example, work your chest and back (pushups) before your arms (bicep curls). Why should you care? Exercises for the larger muscle groups require more energy and utilize the smaller muscle groups during the movement. If you fatigue the smaller muscles first, it will be difficult to do your best on exercises that use the larger muscle groups.

■ Intensity—Lifting too much weight can lead to injury, but lifting weights that are not challenging enough means you probably won't get the results you want. There are several ways to design your strength training program, but a simple test can determine whether you are using the appropriate weight for any given exercise. If you feel like you could keep going when you get to the last two repetitions of your final set, you need to use a heavier weight next time; if you can't complete the number of repetitions and sets you've planned with good form, you need to use a lighter weight. (Hey, no one said this is rocket science, here.)

■ Rest—Avoid strength training the same muscle group(s) on consecutive days. In other words, if you decide to do exercises for your lower body on Monday, wait until Wednesday to do them again. Some people like to do full body strength training routines a couple to three times a week (Monday, Wednesday, and Saturday); others prefer to alternate muscle groups each day (lower body one day, upper body the next, and so on). The rest period enables your muscles to recover from the challenge of training and become stronger over time.

■ Be a smooth operator—Any time you're performing a strength training exercise, use smooth, controlled movements; it's easy to go a little faster and let momentum carry some of the load, but you won't be getting the full benefit unless you allow your muscle to bear all the weight—that goes for the eccentric and concentric portions of the exercise!

■ Include all your muscle groups—Many beginners make the mistake of training only one set of opposing muscle groups (training the abdominal muscles, but not the low back muscles, for example) and wind up with aches, pains, or injuries due to muscular imbalances. Figure 12.1 can help you visualize the major muscle groups. If you aren't sure whether your program hits each group, get help from a certified fitness professional!

FIGURE 12.1

Major muscle groups.

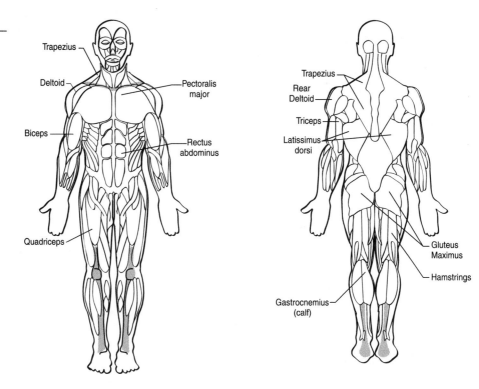

Developing a Strength Training Program

There are literally hundreds of exercises you can do to train the major muscle groups, but for simplicity's sake, you're just going to get a feel for the kind of movement needed to train each group in this chapter. The figures in the following sections illustrate strength exercises you can perform using simple hand weights, but keep in mind that any time you're performing a similar movement (regardless of what provides the resistance), you will be working the same muscle group. You can use your own body weight; resistance bands, balls, and tubing; weight machines; and medicine balls for resistance. Really creative people use soup cans, books, household objects, and even kids and pets (Okay, be safe here, folks—consult a fitness professional before bringing Jimmy or Fido into the mix).

Lunge

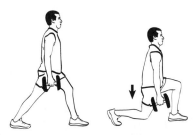

Objective: To strengthen your hamstrings, quadriceps, and gluteal muscles.

1. Hold weights in your hands.
2. Step forward and bend your knees until you're in a lunge position.
3. Lower your trunk toward the floor by slowly bending at the knees to 90 degrees.
4. Return to the original position and repeat with your other leg.

Standing Calf Raise

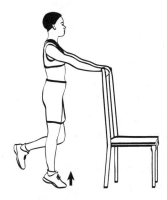

Objective: To strengthen the gastrocnemius.

1. Stand, using a chair for balance if needed.
2. Rise up onto the ball of your right foot.
3. Return to the original position and repeat the desired number of repetitions.
4. Repeat with the other leg.

Modified Push-Up

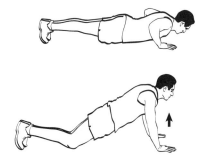

Objective: To strengthen the pectoralis.

1. Begin on the floor by placing your hands slightly wider than shoulder width apart.
2. Push up, keeping your knees on the floor, extending to straight elbows.
3. Maintain a straight back.
4. Lower, so that your upper arms are parallel with the floor, and repeat.

Bent Over Row

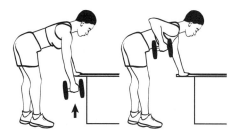

Objective: To strengthen the latissimus dorsi.

1. Slightly bend forward at the hips while maintaining a straight back.
2. Support your upper body with your other arm as shown.
3. Lift your arm up, raising the elbow to shoulder height.
4. Return to the starting position and repeat.

Lateral Raise

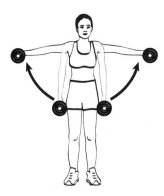

Objective: To strengthen the medial (middle) deltoid.

1. Stand with your feet shoulder width apart and knees slightly bent.
2. With your palms facing inward, lift your arms up and out to the side to shoulder level.
3. Lower the weight and repeat.

Tricep Kickback

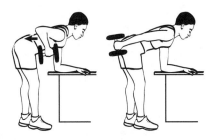

Objective: To strengthen the triceps.

1. Flex at your hip (do not round out the back) leaning over the chair or table.
2. Raise your elbow so that the upper arm is parallel with the floor and close to your body.
3. Use your other arm to maintain balance.
4. Start with the weight directly below the elbow.
5. Extend your arm at the elbow until the arm is straight.
6. Return to the starting position and repeat.

Standing Bicep Curl

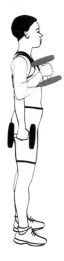

Objective: To strengthen the biceps.

1. Keeping your upper arms close to your side, bend at the elbow and raise the weight to your shoulders.
2. Return to a straight arm position and repeat.
3. Maintain your upper arm in the same position throughout the movement.

Prone Lower Back Extension

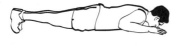

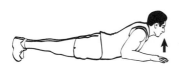

Objective: To strengthen the lower back.

1. Lie face down, elbows bent, arms relaxed and resting on the floor.
2. Arch your back to a comfortable position and hold, keeping the arms relaxed throughout the movement.
3. Return to the starting position and repeat.

Abdominal Crunch

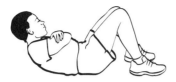

Objective: To strengthen the rectus abdominis.

1. Lie on your back, knees bent, arms crossed over your chest.
2. Lift up your head and continue to lift your shoulders off the floor, toward your knees.
3. Keep your lower back in contact with the floor.
4. Return to the starting position slowly, maintaining the contraction, and repeat.

You're also going to have to figure out how much time you want to devote to strength training in general; how many sets and repetitions you want to perform; and how often you are going to perform the exercises. Let's look at each of these factors individually.

First things first—how much time do you want to spend on strength training? If the answer is, "the bare minimum," you'll need to choose exercises that work a lot of muscle groups at the same time. Think lunges, which use your quadriceps (thighs), gluteus maximus (buttocks), and many other supporting muscles, instead of leg extensions (which focus on quadriceps only). For your upper body, you might choose to do pushups and a bent over row and skip the bicep curls and tricep extensions. Is this optimal? No. Is it efficient, effective, and practical? Yes! Better to do a little strength training than none at all. On the other hand, if you really enjoy strength training and can afford to spend a little more time on it, you might want to look into other resources to help you design a challenging, effective program that meets your needs.

A second important consideration is the number of sets and repetitions you intend to perform. Sets first—if you're new to strength training, start with one set of each exercise. When that no longer feels challenging, see whether you can perform two sets. You can probably see further gains in strength and endurance by adding a third set, but it won't make a dramatic difference. Now reps—if you'd really like to work on muscle strength as opposed to muscle endurance, try using more resistance (heavier weights) and lifting them fewer times (6 to 8 repetitions). If you're focusing on muscle toning and endurance, try using less resistance and performing more repetitions (12 to 15—if you can do more than 15 repetitions, you probably need to increase the weight). If your goal is simply to become healthier and more fit, you can go somewhere in the middle—perform 8 to 12 repetitions using a challenging, but moderate, weight. If the last two repetitions of your program feel easy, it's time to increase the weight (or resistance).

Finally, you need to determine how often you will strength train. If you have four days per week to sneak in a little routine, you can successfully divide your exercises into categories such as upper and lower body. On Monday, you might do exercises for your chest, back, shoulders, arms, abdominals, and low back. On Tuesday, you can do exercises for your thighs, hamstrings, buttocks, and calves. On Wednesday, you might like a day off; then Thursday, you can repeat Monday's upper body routine and Friday is another lower body routine. On the other hand, if you only want to strength train two or three days per week, you'll need to do a full body routine each day (exercises for all the major muscle groups Monday and Thursday or Monday, Wednesday, and Saturday, for example).

Developing an effective strength training routine can really make all the difference in your energy level, your appearance, and the way you feel in your own skin. Unfortunately, strength training myths abound. Keep reading to make sure you aren't falling victim to urban legends!

Common Myths and Misconceptions

Can I work out consistently at first and then train every once in a while to maintain my muscle strength and endurance?

No. As with any other aspect of fitness, strength returns to near pretraining levels without consistent exercise. Studies do show that this process takes a little longer with muscle strength and endurance than with cardiovascular fitness, but why get behind? It is much easier to keep up than to catch up!

I am a woman and don't want to "bulk up." Can I still strength train?

Yes! Most women cannot develop bulky muscles because they have low levels of testosterone, a hormone required for building muscle mass. They can, however, gain muscle strength and endurance without gaining a lot of muscle mass. If you tend to gain muscle mass easily (and there are some women out there who do) and you'd prefer not to, try lifting lighter weights and increase your repetitions. This will help minimize an increase in muscle size and mass, while still providing the overall benefits of strength training.

Can I turn my fat into muscle with training?

No. Muscle and fat are physiologically distinct tissues. One can never "turn into" the other. If you begin a strength training program, get regular cardiovascular exercise, and eat well, you may be able to reduce your fat stores and increase your muscle mass, but the opposite is also true. When people stop training, their fat stores may increase because they are no longer burning as many calories, and muscle mass, strength, and endurance may decrease due to a lack of conditioning.

Can I target a specific area for fat loss?

No. People are genetically prone to storing fat in certain areas. Exercises targeted at these areas can strengthen the muscles but will not eliminate fat from the area. The only way to lose fat is to consistently burn more calories than you consume (see Chapter 4, "Balanced Nutrition"), but this still doesn't guarantee that you'll be able to reduce fat in specific areas. Focus on your health, include cardiovascular and strength training, and eat plenty of satisfying, nutrient-rich meals and snacks—let nature take care of the rest!

Will I lose flexibility if I strength train?

Not if you move through a full range of motion during each exercise and remember to include some stretching as part of your overall exercise plan. Stretch the worked muscles between sets to incorporate flexibility exercises into your regular strength training routine.

THE ABSOLUTE MINIMUM

- Strength training builds muscle mass, strength, and endurance and helps maintain bone health.
- Incorporate two to three full-body strength workouts per week to get the maximum benefit—be sure to hit all your major muscle groups.
- Progression, progression, progression. Got it? Begin slowly with both cardiovascular and strength training to avoid injury and burnout.
- Don't stress over doing it perfectly—just get out there and give it a shot!

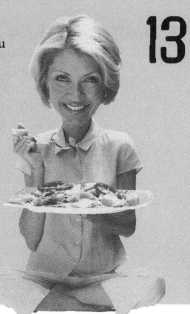

13

EXERCISING AT HOME AND ON THE ROAD

Although fitness centers are ideal for providing support, motivation, feedback, and an all-weather location for exercise, it's important to realize that many options for exercise are available in the comfort and convenience of your own home. For those of you who travel frequently, or are concerned that an upcoming vacation will sideline your fitness routine, take heart—with the right attitude, equipment, and a few simple guidelines, you can stay fit on the road, too!

Building a "Home Gym"

Many people choose to designate a room or an area of their homes for fitness equipment and exercise. Basements and rec rooms work wonderfully for this purpose, but a mat and some floor space are truly all you need. After you've chosen an appropriate space, decide whether you require or desire additional equipment, considering your fitness level, budget, and time constraints before you go gung ho into the nearest fitness equipment retail store. All the following are *possibilities*, but not necessities, in terms of home fitness equipment:

- Traditional stationary equipment—Treadmills, bikes, rowing machines, stair climbers, and elliptical trainers can all provide significant cardiovascular benefits when used properly and consistently. Be sure to *test* the equipment before buying, and check that it comes with a warranty. Because these pieces usually involve a pretty significant financial investment, do your homework and research the equipment with *Consumer Reports* before buying. Be sure you feel comfortable operating the equipment and understanding the display panel. See the following section, "A Primer on Home Fitness Equipment," for more information on selecting an appropriate piece of cardiovascular equipment.

note

Cardiovascular equipment display panels often include calorie expenditure estimates. These numbers typically overestimate true energy expenditure, so don't get hung up on them or try to use them to calculate your total daily calorie needs. You're not supposed to be obsessed with calories anyway, right?

    Cheap alternatives: Use your stairwell for an intense aerobic workout or for providing short bursts of activity for a circuit-type workout; jumping rope is also a huge calorie-burner (make sure that you have plenty of room, or just use an imaginary rope); when weather permits, brisk walking is one of the best all-around choices for health. If weather or safety becomes an issue, try walking at your local mall. Whenever I spent the night at my grandparents' house as a kid (okay, sometimes as a young adult, too), one of my favorite activities was mall walking with Grandma.

- Home strength training equipment—Follow the same guidelines as with traditional cardio equipment. Research the product before buying, test it if possible, and make sure that it is sold under warranty and includes safety features.

Cheap alternatives: Resistance bands or tubing, hand weights, and stability balls are effective strength training tools available at most major retail stores; see the sample exercises at the end of the chapter that use resistance tubing for a total body strength training routine. *Really* frugal exercisers use items around the house or their own body weight for resistance! Fill a clean gallon milk jug with water, and you've got an 8-pound weight; fill it half full for 4 pounds if you're just embarking on a strength training program. Use the weight of your own body in exercises such as push-ups, abdominal crunches, tricep dips, lunges, and toe raises.

▓ Exercise videos—These little fitness gems can be used for cardio, strength, and flexibility training and provide the advantage of a low-pressure introduction to new exercise skills. However, it is challenging to assess your own form and technique without personal attention from an instructor. You may want to try a group fitness class geared toward beginners first, and then move on to videos.

Cheap alternatives: Borrow videos from your local library or rent them from a video store to prevent boredom. Another low-cost option is to start a video swap with co-workers, friends, relatives, or neighbors.

A Primer on Home Fitness Equipment

How many of us have expensive "clothes racks" in our bedrooms, basements, and rec rooms because we simply don't utilize home fitness equipment as we'd hoped? Avoid this mistake (or don't make it twice!) by familiarizing yourself with the advantages and disadvantages of some of the most popular pieces of cardiovascular equipment available for use in your home.

Stationary bikes (upright or recumbent):

▓ Excellent choice for heavier individuals and beginners.

▓ Low-impact movement is ideal for people with a history of low back problems or joint pain.

▓ Relatively inexpensive.

▓ Require less space than many other pieces.

▓ Two basic models—upright bikes simulate outdoor cycling and tend to cost less; recumbent bikes provide a more relaxed, extended position and more comfortable seats, and are easier to mount and dismount for people with limited mobility.

▓ Resistance can be provided by friction (cheapest), air (moderately priced), and magnets (most expensive and highest quality).

Treadmills:

- Easier on joints than walking/running on pavement.
- Encourage high energy expenditure due to weight-bearing nature of the movement.
- Look for models that allow you to choose the incline—set at 4% or greater to better simulate walking/running outside.
- Nonmotorized models *not* recommended—check for warranty on motorized models.
- Test the equipment to make sure it accommodates your walking and running stride.
- May require more space than other pieces of equipment.
- Look for models with safety handles and emergency stop features.

Rowing machines:

- Simulate outdoor rowing; resistance provided by air or water—the harder you pull, the higher the resistance.
- Works lower *and* upper body muscle groups.
- Low-impact movement ideal for heavier people and beginners.
- May not be comfortable for people with a history of low back pain/injury.
- Look for machines that offer smooth, even resistance throughout the movement and a comfortable, non-slip seat.
- Models with adjustable, pivoting foot plates allow for greater comfort.
- Educate yourself on proper rowing technique before use, or have a fitness professional evaluate your technique in person.

Elliptical trainers:

- Simulate a cross between running and climbing; feet create an elliptical pattern during the movement.
- Some models offer upper-body resistance with "poles" that coordinate with leg movements.
- Can be used in reverse to stimulate different muscle groups in the lower body.
- Provide a low-impact, high-intensity alternative to walking/running.
- Tend to require more space, coordination, balance, and practice.
- May be costly for high-quality models.

Stair climbers:

- Resistance via air, hydraulic, or magnetic brakes—hydraulic or magnetic brakes are preferred, and magnetic brakes offer the smoothest movement.
- Offer high-intensity, low-impact workouts.
- Some models utilize foot plates that operate independently—both can be up or down at the same time. Others utilize dependent foot plates—when one goes down, the other automatically goes up (nice for beginners, but doesn't provide the same level of intensity).
- Require a little more coordination and skill than some other types of equipment.

Maintaining Motivation

One of the most challenging aspects of working out at home is maintaining motivation. Sometimes, home exercise is almost too convenient. If your "home gym" is located near the kitchen, dining room, office, bedroom, or living room, you may be tempted to eat, pay bills, relax, sleep, or watch TV instead of exercising as planned. Other people have no trouble tuning out the demands at home and view time spent in their workout "zone" as an investment in their health and well being. The key is in knowing yourself. If you've purchased every piece of exercise equipment ever featured in an infomercial and haven't yet been able to incorporate one of them into a regular exercise routine, it's possible that home fitness just isn't your bag. You're not a failure; you just haven't found your niche yet. If that's the case, be honest and start figuring out what does work. Try group fitness classes, fitness centers, personal trainers, mall walking, training for events, or simply increasing daily activity. If you want to give home fitness a fair shot, check out the following section, "Slow and Steady Wins the Race," for a little inspiration, or try the tips in the section "Sticking with It" later in the chapter.

Slow and Steady Wins the Race (Marie's Story)

Marie's (not her real name) story is much like many of yours. She was slim and physically active as a child, but after entering the workforce at a relatively young age, playing took a back burner to school and her job. She gained weight gradually, a couple of pounds every year, until she wound up with debilitating knee pain in 1996 at the age of 44. An MRI confirmed that she had arthritis and that both knee caps pulled to the outside, which was making even walking extremely difficult. After two knee surgeries, one in 1996 and another in 1998, Marie had all but given up on any form of physical activity. Her condition made it painful to move, and her lack of activity contributed to additional weight gain. In 2000, she had exploratory surgery on her knees again to determine whether any other procedures might help, but her doctor explained that they had done all they could. And that was the day that Marie decided to act:

"I could tell it wasn't good. I knew I needed to do something, so I decided to walk the 5K race that's part of the Indianapolis 500 Festival Mini Marathon. I bought the NIFS manual and participated that year."

It wasn't a smooth journey. Marie readily admits that she got sidelined many times with illness or other responsibilities, but she kept at it. By the time she participated in the NIFS/Clarian Women's LivLite Advantage program in 2002, she felt truly ready to lose weight:

"I had tried other programs before, but you always had to count something or weigh foods. I learned that I can eat what I want and know that, in the long run, it's fine. I lost 35 pounds, and I've been steady at my current weight for about four months. I've decided that's okay. I was wearing [size] 24's and now I'm wearing 16's, and it feels so good."

Marie discovered things about herself that she never would have dreamed:

"I really like sweating! It means I've worked my body, and that's how it lets me know. I've discovered new fruits and vegetables that I truly enjoy eating, and my body lets me know when I haven't done a good job with drinking my eight glasses of water a day."

She admits it's not always easy and gives much credit to her close friend and exercise buddy and other supportive people for helping her stay on track, but she's found ways to make it work, little by little. When it's too difficult to get to the fitness center, Marie has an alternative:

"I have an elliptical machine at home, and I have a little aerobics routine. I usually have the TV or radio on, and I do 20 or 25 minutes [of cardiovascular activity]. I also have a resistance ball and stretchy bands for strength training. I might spend 60 minutes or more on the weekends just doing my own thing at home."

When asked whether she had any advice for readers contemplating making these same lifestyle changes, Marie emphasized moderation:

"Drastic changes don't work. If you can't eat your favorite foods, it simply doesn't stick. You can do that for a while, but you always go back to your favorites. You have to want it for yourself, deep inside, or you won't be able to work as hard as you have to. And it is hard work. I may have to do more to continue seeing the results I want, but I don't want to do it quickly, because that kind of weight loss doesn't stick, and I want this to be permanent."

Well put, Marie!

Sticking with It

The following are tips for staying consistent with home exercise:

- Exercise early—Because so many distractions crop up at home, morning tends to be the best time to schedule your workout.

- Lay out your shoes and exercise clothing the night before; get a water bottle and sweat towel ready, too.

- Make your home fitness area more appealing by placing equipment near a television or radio, stocking a shelf with good reading material, and providing adequate lighting; a fan and good ventilation help you stay comfortable and healthy.

- Schedule your home workout just like any other appointment—write it in your planner or on a wall calendar.

- Create a home fitness "challenge"—each person in your household tracks his or her exercise time on a wall calendar with colored stickers; determine age- and budget-appropriate prizes for the monthly winner.

- Meet with a personal trainer to develop or revise your home fitness routine; this health professional can ensure that you get the best results for your time and effort.

Fitness on the Go

Many people who travel frequently for business or pleasure find it difficult to maintain consistency in their exercise routines. There's no question that it takes some effort to squeeze exercise into busy conference and meeting schedules or once in a lifetime sight-seeing trips, so the first thing you need to assess is how big a role travel fitness will play in your overall fitness routine.

If you travel once a year for a major two-week vacation, you don't need to be fanatic about structured exercise. In fact, your body just might appreciate a little break. Plan active vacations when possible by researching hiking, biking, or walking tours of your destination—there's no better way to experience the true culture and flavor of another area! Even if you don't participate in a fitness-minded tour, do your best to walk as much as possible to maintain a minimal level of activity. More importantly, schedule a workout for the day after you return, perhaps with a friend or personal trainer for a little built-in accountability. It isn't the inactivity *during* the vacation that gets most people off track—it's the inability to get back into a consistent pattern after they get home.

If, on the other hand, you travel several days to a week or more out of each month, it makes sense to stick to your normal routine as closely as possible. You have the more difficult job, but with a little planning and effort, you really can take your healthy habits on the road. Use the following techniques if you're a frequent traveler:

- Do some research—By planning ahead, you can make sure that fitness doesn't take a back burner on your trip. Surf the Internet or call your hotel well in advance to scope out your destination. Does your hotel offer an onsite fitness facility or pool? Are parks, walking paths, sidewalks, or beaches nearby? Can you rent a bike, paddleboat, or rollerblades to check out the local offerings? Be sure to get your hotel staff's recommendations regarding the safety of the area before you strike out on your own in unfamiliar surroundings.

- Pack early—A few days before you leave, pack your exercise tools in a nylon stuff bag to keep everything in one place and handy to throw into your suitcase or carry-on. Most of these items are available at your local sporting goods store, fitness center, or major retail store. Remember to pack the following:

  - Walking shoes
  - Lightweight, comfortable exercise clothing
  - Bathing suit
  - Your favorite fitness video
  - Resistance bands or tubing
  - Collapsible hand weights that can be filled with water
  - Jump rope
  - Magazines, books, or headphones for making your stationary bike ride a little more interesting

- Do a condensed, intense workout—Time is usually at a premium on the road, so it may behoove you to crank up the intensity a bit and exercise for a shorter length of time. If you normally ride a stationary bike for 45 minutes at a moderate intensity, try doing 20 minutes with extra resistance. Another option is doing a circuit workout by incorporating short bursts of high-intensity aerobic exercise into your travel strength training routine. Try doing

30 to 45 seconds of jumping rope, jumping jacks, or stair climbing between each strength training set. This type of workout keeps your heart rate elevated much more so than traditional strength training, so you can consider it a cardiovascular and strength session all in one.

■ Rehearse your routine—You want a travel workout that's simple and automatic—so practice it! Be comfortable with your exercises before you have to do them without an instructor. See the following section, "Sample Home or Travel Resistance Exercises," for a simple routine to get you started.

■ Try airport exercise—So you've got a 2-hour layover? Pack or wear walking or running shoes and use the extra time to walk the terminals. Avoiding escalators and automated walking bridges will also help you burn a few extra calories. During the flight, get up and walk the length of the plane as often as possible to keep your blood circulating and to reduce the risk of deep vein thrombosis (DVT). See the following sidebar for more information.

DEEP VEIN *WHAT*?!

Deep vein thrombosis (DVT) is a serious condition caused when a blood clot forms in the lower extremities. This condition can be fatal if the clot breaks loose and travels to the lungs, blocking the pulmonary artery. There are many risk factors for DVT, but travelers who remain immobile for long flights or car trips are especially vulnerable and should take the following precautions:

■ Walk briskly or exercise shortly before leaving.

■ Dress in comfortable, loose clothing—slip out of your shoes after departure and put on a pair of warm, dry socks to encourage good circulation.

■ Bring a water bottle and avoid alcoholic beverages—dehydration doesn't help anyone.

■ Stop at rest areas frequently, or get up and walk the length of the plane every hour.

■ Do some simple stretches in your seat. Rotate your ankles, shift your weight, and tighten and release muscles in your lower body.

■ Talk with your doctor about compression socks—these may be appropriate if you have other risk factors.

■ Plan to relax—Don't expect relaxation to happen automatically while you're traveling. Bring a few items from home that help you unwind after long days and weeks—decaffeinated tea bags, CDs with soft music or relaxation scripts, comfy sleepwear, and so on. Try gentle stretching and deep breathing before you go to bed—many people have good intentions to exercise while traveling but give up because they're just too tired.

Sample Home or Travel Resistance Exercises

The following sections describe some sample resistance exercises you can do at home or on the road.

For a circuit workout, after you warm up, move through the following exercises, performing one or two sets of 12 repetitions each, doing 30 to 45 seconds of higher intensity cardiovascular activity between each exercise. Jumping jacks, jumping rope (real or imaginary!), or stair climbing are simple indoor options for your cardio "bursts."

Arm Curl

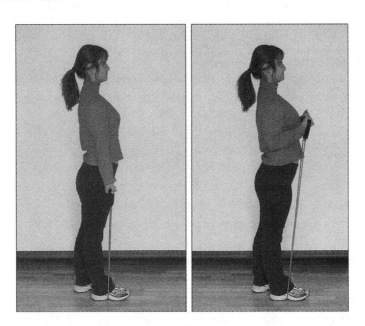

Muscle Group: Biceps

1. Stand on the center of the resistance tube with the tubing under the arch of one or both feet.

2. Hold the resistance tube handles at your sides with arms extended. Palms are facing away from your body.

3. Keep the upper arms at your side and bend the elbows to bring palms up toward the shoulders.

4. Slowly extend the arms back to the start position at your sides and repeat.

Arm Extension

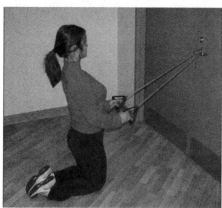 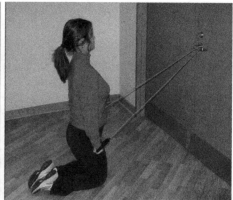

Muscle Group: Triceps

1. Wrap the resistance tube around both doorknobs of an open door or a fixed handle as shown above.

2. Kneel on the ground facing the door and grasp the handles with palms facing the floor.

3. Keep the upper arms stationary against the body and bend the elbows.

4. Slowly extend the arms by straightening the elbows as you push the forearms downward. Palms should face behind you.

5. Slowly release to starting position and repeat.

Single-Arm Front Raise

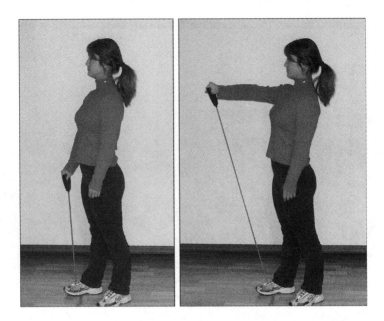

Muscle Group: Anterior deltoid (the front part of your shoulder)

1. Stand with the resistance tube securely under the arch of both feet.
2. Hold the handle of the resistance tube with the arm down at your side.
3. With palm facing down, slowly extend the arm upward to shoulder height.
4. Slowly lower and repeat. Perform the exercise on the opposite arm.

Side Raise

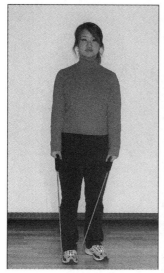 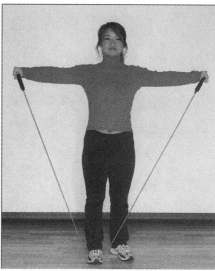

Muscle Group: Medial deltoid (the middle of your shoulder)

1. Stand on the center of the resistance tube with the tubing under the arch of one foot.

2. Grasp the handles with arms down at your sides. (Note: This exercise can be performed as a single-arm raise.)

3. Raise arm out to the sides, up to shoulder height. The palms of your hands should face the floor.

4. Slowly bring arms back down to starting position and repeat.

Chest Press

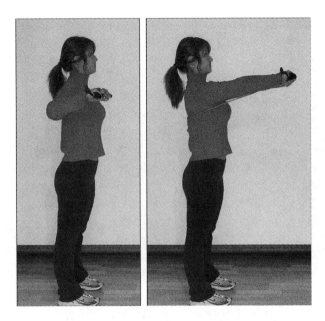

Muscle Group: Pectoralis major (your chest)

1. Stand with feet hip-distance apart.
2. Place the resistance tubing around your upper back and grip handles with palms facing forward. (Note: You may wrap an extra length of the resistance tubing around your hands to increase tension.)
3. Start with the elbows at a 90-degree angle and extend arms forward.
4. Slowly return to starting position and repeat.

Modified Push-Up/Traditional Push-Up

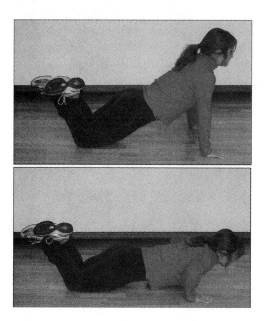

(Modified push-up pictured.)

Muscle Group: Pectoralis major (chest muscles again; great for the entire upper body)

1. Place hands on the floor, slightly wider than shoulder-width apart. Arms are extended.

2. Knees are bent and on the floor for the modified push-up. For the traditional push-up, the legs are straight, and the body is supported up on the toes.

3. Bend elbows and lower the chest toward the floor.

4. Slowly extend arms straight back to starting position.

Rear Delt Fly

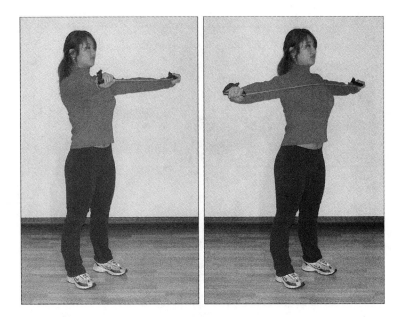

Muscle Group: Posterior deltoid (back of your shoulder)

1. Stand with feet hip-distance apart.
2. Grasp handles and wrap the resistance tubing around your hands for appropriate tension.
3. Raise arms in front to shoulder height and width.
4. Pull arms out toward your sides as the resistance tubing is pulled across your chest.
5. Slowly release the cord back to the starting position and repeat.

Standing Row

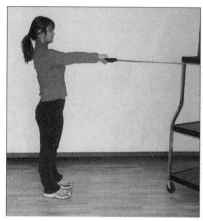 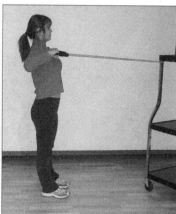

Muscle Group: Posterior deltoid, Trapezius (back of your shoulder and upper back)

1. This exercise requires that the resistance tubing is secured around a sturdy, nonmovable post.

2. Begin by wrapping the resistance tubing around the post at midchest height.

3. Grasp the handles and let your arms extend straight out in front of your body. Palms are facing the floor.

4. Pull both handles back toward your body, squeezing your shoulder blades together. Elbows are bent and slightly behind your body.

5. Slowly extend arms back to starting position and repeat.

Abdominal Curl

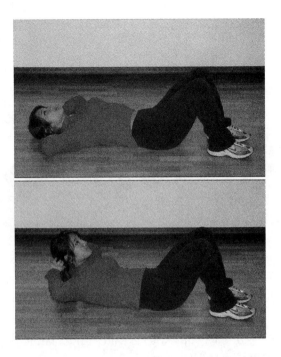

Muscle Group: Rectus abdominus (work those stomach muscles)

1. Lie on your back with knees bent and feet flat on the floor.

2. Place your hands lightly on the back of your head with elbows out to the side.

3. Raise the shoulder blades off the floor and exhale as you contract the abdominal muscles.

4. Slowly lower back to starting position and repeat.

Reverse Curl

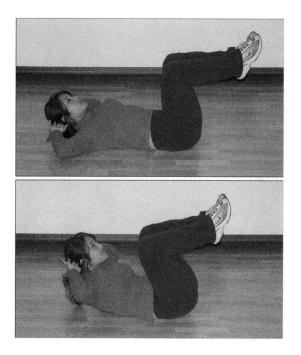

Muscle Group: Rectus abdominus

1. Lie on your back with elbows out to the side. Hips are flexed and knees are bent at a 90-degree angle.

2. Slowly bring the knees in toward the chest. At the same time, use the abdominal muscles to lift the shoulder blades off the floor.

3. Slowly return to starting position and repeat.

Standing Lunge

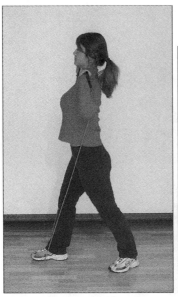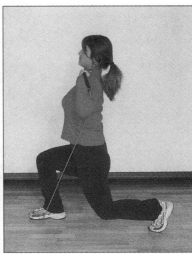

Muscle Groups: Quadriceps, Gluteals, Hamstrings

1. Place the center of the resistance band securely under one foot.

2. Stand upright with elbows bent, holding the handles of the resistance band stationary at shoulder height.

3. Take a large step backward with the leg that is not stepping on the band.

4. The back leg is supported on the ball of that foot, and the knee of the front foot should form a 90-degree angle with the ankle.

5. Keeping the chest up, slowly bend the back knee until a 90-degree angle is formed with the back leg.

6. Slowly straighten the knees to starting position and repeat. Perform the same exercise on the opposite leg.

Single-Leg Curl

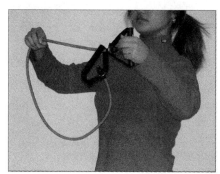
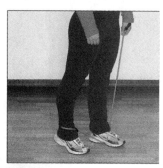
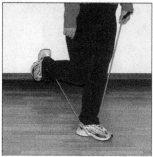

Muscle Group: Hamstrings

1. Feed one end of the resistance tube through the other handle to form a loop.
2. Place the loop around one ankle. Step on the excess band length with the other foot and hold onto the handle.
3. Keeping the thigh stationary, bend the knee so that the foot curls up toward the glutes.
4. Slowly lower and repeat. Perform the same exercise on the opposite leg.

THE ABSOLUTE MINIMUM

- Know thyself! Is home fitness a realistic option for you at this time in your life?

- If yes, dedicate a particular area of your home to exercise and equipment, and make it as pleasant as possible.

- Research any piece of equipment thoroughly and test it in person before buying—make sure it comes with a warranty.

- Invest in some small, inexpensive pieces for home strength training, such as stability balls, hand weights, or resistance tubing.

- Get advice about setting up a home fitness program from a knowledgeable, certified fitness professional.

- Plan ahead for traveling, but don't get bent out of shape if you can't do 100% of your normal routine.

- Emphasize *movement*, not just *exercise*, as much as possible when traveling and life makes it difficult to be structured.

- Relax, enjoy yourself and your new lifestyle, and be fully present in every moment!

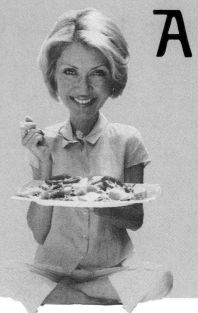

A

WORKSHEETS AND ADDITIONAL RESOURCES

Blood Lipid Classifications*

Total Cholesterol (mg/dl)

< 200	Desirable
200 to 239	Borderline High
≥ 240	High

LDL Cholesterol (mg/dl)

< 100	Optimal
100 to 129	Near Optimal
130 to 159	Borderline High
160 to 189	High
≥ 190	Very High

HDL Cholesterol (mg/dl)

< 40	Low
≥ 60	High

Triglycerides (mg/dl)

< 150	Normal
150 to 199	Borderline High
200 to 499	High
≥ 500	Very High

*Adapted from the *Third Report of the National Cholesterol Education Program (NCEP) Expert Panel on Detection, Evaluation, and Treatment of High Blood Cholesterol in Adults*; NIH Publication No. 01-3670, May 2001.

Blood Pressure (BP) Classifications (mm/Hg)**

Systolic BP	Diastolic BP	Classification
< 120	and < 80	Normal
120 to 139	or 80 to 89	Prehypertension
140 to 159	or 90 to 99	Stage 1 Hypertension
≥ 160	or ≥ 100	Stage 2 Hypertension

**Adapted from the *7th Report of the Joint National Committee on Prevention, Detection, Evaluation, and Treatment of High Blood Pressure*; NIH Publication No. 03-5233, May 2003.

Fasting Blood Glucose (mg/dL)***

< 100	Normal
100 to 126	Impaired Fasting Glucose (indicates "prediabetes" in nondiabetics)
≥ 126	Indicates need for retesting to diagnose diabetes

***Adapted from *Diabetes Care* 27:S11-S14, 2004.

Worksheets

Figures A.1, A.2, and A.3 show worksheets that you can use to log your daily food choices, weekly activity choices, and weekly goals and action steps, respectively. All three of these worksheets are available for download as printable PDFs from the Que website. Go to http://www.quepublishing.com/ and type this book's ISBN (0789733153) into the Search field to go to this book's web page. You can download the PDFs from there.

FIGURE A.1

Daily food choices.

Daily Food Choices

Date: _____   Day of week: _____

Time	Hunger/Fullness Rating Pre-Meal/Post-Meal	Amount	Food or Beverage	Location	Feelings

Goals:

Challenges:

for every body.

nifs

National Institute

FIGURE A.2

Weekly activity choices.

Weekly Activity Choices

Week of _____

Date/Time	Type of Activity	Length of Activity	Level of Difficulty	Heart Rate (optional)	Feelings

Goals:

Challenges:

FIGURE A.3
Weekly goals and action steps.

Weekly Goals and Action Steps

for every body.
nifs
National Institute for Fitness and Sport

Week of ________________

My long term goal(s) is/are:

My short term goal(s) is/are:

This week, I plan on taking the following action steps in order to meet my short term goal(s):

Last week, I learned the following about myself:

Some of the challenges I faced last week were:

Potential strategies for each of these challenges include:

Recommended Reading

The Intrinsic Exerciser: Discovering the Joy of Exercise by Jay Kimiecik, Houghton Mifflin Company, 2002.

Fit from Within: 101 Simple Secrets to Change Your Body and Your Life—Starting Today and Lasting Forever by Victoria Moran, McGraw-Hill, 2002.

Intuitive Eating: A Revolutionary Program That Works by Evelyn Tribole and Elyse Resch, St. Martin's Griffin, 2nd Edition, 2003.

Secrets of Feeding a Healthy Family by Ellyn Satter, Kelcy Press, 1999.

Child of Mine: Feeding with Love and Good Sense by Ellyn Satter, Bull Publishing Company, 3rd Edition, 2000.

How to Get Your Kid to Eat...But Not Too Much by Ellyn Satter, Bull Publishing Company, 1987.

Index

How can we make this index more useful? Email us at indexes@quepublishing.com

How can we make this index more useful? Email us at indexes@quepublishing.com

How can we make this index more useful? Email us at indexes@quepublishing.com

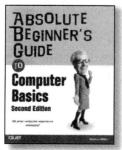
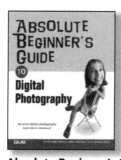
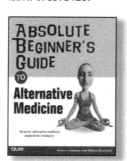
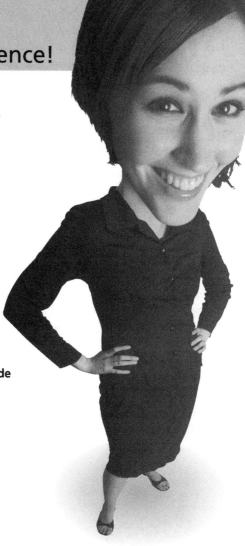
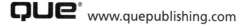

Do Even More
...In No Time

Get ready to cross off those items on your to-do list! *In No Time* helps you tackle the projects that you don't think you have time to finish. With shopping lists and step-by-step instructions, these books get you working toward accomplishing your goals.

Check out these other *In No Time* books, coming soon!

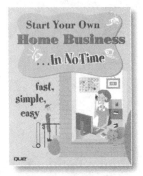

Start Your Own Home Business In No Time
ISBN: **0-7897-3224-6**
$16.95
September 2004

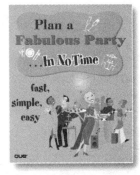

Plan a Fabulous Party In No Time
ISBN: **0-7897-3221-1**
$16.95
November 2004

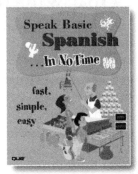

Speak Basic Spanish In No Time
ISBN: **0-7897-3223-8**
$16.95
September 2004

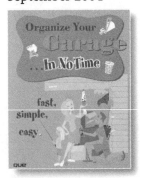

Organize Your Garage In No Time
ISBN: **0-7897-3219-X**
$16.95
February 2005

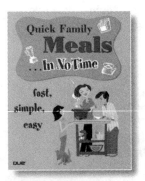

Quick Family Meals In No Time
ISBN: **0-7897-3299-8**
$16.95
October 2004

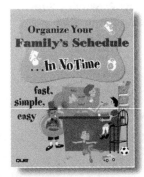

Organize Your Family's Schedule In No Time
ISBN: **0-7897-3220-3**
$16.95
October 2004